T0282697

This book offers more than a few stories. It offers practical advice on how to care for women as soon as fistula develops. It also acts as a prompt for deeper discussions on how to support women holistically. For those who are not aware of the consequences of obstetric fistula to women, this book can be extremely upsetting. I say this to manage expectations, not to deter people from reading it. It is a powerful, and essential book for everyone including clinicians, psychologists and social scientists working in sexual and reproductive healthcare, maternal health policy makers and educationalists. I hope this book is read widely by those from varying disciplines.

Professor Dame Tina Lavender
Professor of Maternal and Newborn Health
The Liverpool School of Tropical Medicine
UK

Acknowledgments

We wish to thank all women who have broken the fistula secrecy to access care services in designated centres. Their willingness and desire to serve as community volunteers is truly inspirational. This book could not have seen the light of day without their stories as we journeyed with each one of them through their care.

Our gratitude goes to Jessey and Alex for recreating parts of the narratives. In addition, we would like to thank Naima at Moran (E. A.) Publishers: her motivation and technical support has made publishing this book a dream come true.

Dedication

This book is dedicated to every woman experiencing fistula following child birth – your resilience and determination to overcome the shame and rejection is truly amazing.

To our children, Vanessa, Frank and Alvin, your compassion, understanding and witty nature gives your parents peace, pride and freedom to serve others.

Preface

This book presents the lived experiences of women living with fistula before and after surgery. It is written in narrative form and intended for every person with a heart to love and be loved. The authors present captivating stories of women who journeyed with fistula in their private and public lives.

We hope that our readers will drink our passion and join the conversation that will help bring to an end a chapter that should never have been written for women anywhere on planet Earth.

$$Part_1$$

Stories narrated by the victims

—••●•••—

Personal Perspectives on Obstetric Fistula and Stillbirth

Background

The story of obstetric fistula reads like a bad dream. It is one of those conditions that can easily be looked at as unjust and unfair. Yet, stakeholders maintain a studious silence despite the fact that health-related issues like obstetric fistula fall squarely at the centre of community interest, albeit negatively. Commonly, women with fistula experience loss of role in their community and family, isolation and economic hardships. Their ability to work, travel and socialize is affected. Majority of these problems result from cultural dynamics and power plays. As a result, these cultural dynamics influence people's behaviour, who in most cases suffer from a general sense of lack of awareness and appreciation of fistula as a medical reality. Based on these societal views, the narratives in this chapter are told by women who lived with fistula before and after surgery.

A Rock and a Hard Place

The journey from Kisumu to Homa Bay was horrible. I was afraid to get to my destination. I could not risk exposing my shameful condition. How would people react when they looked at a big girl who had wetted herself like a mindless child? I had to find a way to alight after everybody had gotten off the bus so that nobody witnessed my mess – that meant that I was going to sit in the vehicle until it arrived at its final destination for me to leave last.

That morning, my husband with whom we lived in the city had escorted me to the bus stage to head to their village in Homa Bay where his parents lived. I felt sad that I would miss him. However, since he had promised to visit every weekend, I was consoled. My joy was also doubled by the thought of his plans to build me a house in the village where he would later move in too. Like the good wife that I was, I submitted and took the bus home as I allowed him enough space to build a financial foundation for the family. I did not know that I would never see him again. The last image I had of him, with bouts of bitterness, was his waving hand bidding me goodbye as the bus crawled out of the station. I waved back, cheerfully and tearfully. I wished I had not.

"Madam, your money ends here!" the conductor arrogantly reminded me.

We were two stages past my destination, but the bus was still full. I was terrified to get up. But since I had no extra money to pay fare, I had to hastily do the walk of shame from the last seat towards the door. I had barely made three steps from my seat when a young child innocently raised its voice to report to the mother that my dress was wet and I was stinking of urine. I hastened my steps, feeling the surprised eyes and faces behind me, thanks to the innocent whistleblower on its mother's laps. The child may have gone on wondering loudly whether urinating on oneself was not a child's forte.

I survived the near panic attack that was the import of my march to exit the bus. While I headed home, I was also entertaining the hope that Mark's parents would find a cure for my humiliating condition. Mark had often related to me that besides his mum's tailoring job, she was an experienced herbalist who could treat anything under the sun. I was full of joy that I was going to stay with my husband's parents. To me, that was a real sign that they had accepted me into their family.

I was however hit by a thunderbolt of shock at their cold reception. Mark's mum struggled to suppress her surprise upon seeing me. His dad greeted me hurriedly, uttered a colourless 'welcome' and got back to his carpentry work as if I was a frequent and common visitor.

"So, you are here…," he said again as an afterthought, a filler for the awkward silence.

"Yes. Mark asked me to come," I responded politely and with a curtsy. He went on with his business almost as if we were not having a conversation. I had met both Mark's father and mother before, but not in such an intense setting.

Mark's mother, who was seated right next to us, expressed overt indifference and lack of warmth, which instantly reminded me of Mark's reaction after my delivery, and for the better part of the six months after delivery as I struggled to understand my new condition.

After what had happened during my first delivery where I had endured the pain of losing a child, I swore never to deliver again in a hospital. Those evil nurses would extend their hurt attitude towards me and my innocent child. I could not stand their big bad eyes and their enormous mouths that would not hesitate to throw grenades of expletives at poor women. They would even go as far as cursing my child. A friend I met at the delivery ward, Sister Sandra, had related to us how she was mistreated for accidentally farting as she received an injection. You would think that they themselves never farted. As that was her sixth delivery at the hospital, one nurse had even told her to stop delivering babies as if she had won a government tender to supply the nation with ugly babies.

When I became pregnant again, the second time, I was excited for now I would redeem my image and give Mark a family. I had just begun experiencing labour, and Mark's relatives, his elder sister and an aunt, who had pitched camp at our two-roomed house assured me that a revered traditional birth attendant would help me deliver safely. The community midwife had created quite a name for herself for successfully handling five deliveries among Mark's relatives.

"*Nyako* (girl), push!" she would command as I seethed in pain.

Everything about her was crude. Her tone was arrogant. Her hands were violent. The pain was unimaginable. I thought that my vaginal walls were bursting, more like a grenade had been dropped between my thighs. In that period, I realized that pain is cold, it is never hot. I had screamed my lungs out and my voice away. Nothing was left but the pain. It shot through every inch of my body.

"Push! Push!" I heard the orders; they infuriated me.

What more did they want me to push, my intestines? I screamed back with overtones of anger and pain.

The process was brutal enough. When it was all done and I could feel that my womb was empty, all I wanted to see was my child, to hold and hear it shoot its first cry. Untraditionally, nobody was congratulating me. Nobody was saying a word. As I surveyed from each of the relative's faces, they had a single tale to tell. Yet they remained silent. I jumped my gaze to that of the revered midwife. She did not hesitate to announce.

"It died!" she said in what sounded like a triumphant voice.

"What died?"

"The thing."

"What thing?" I insisted, demanding a clear answer.

Mark did not speak to me for a week. A woman whose child died at birth was believed to be a bad omen to her husband. I was mourning. My husband was not talking to me. My bladder had suddenly gone loose. The tragedy was threefold. I could no longer control my stool and urine. I would be walking and suddenly urine would escape my panties and trickle down my thighs to the ground. It was overwhelmingly embarrassing.

In addition to the death of our child, which had muted Mark, my new condition further pushed him away. It pained me that I had brought distress to my husband. He was no longer the jovial man he used to be. He was no longer sharing a bed with me. Most times he would fail to return home, three days in a row. Often, I would lie on an empty stomach: I could not eat and I could not stop the pain. I had run out of both my appetite and any energy to fight pain. The community midwife fed me on a variety of herbs which only served to ease my abdominal pains, but did nothing to stop the loss of stool and urine.

While at a church service at some point, despite the many underclothes I had worn to prevent leakage, the unforgiving urine found a way of embarrassing me. I ran out of the church and never showed my face there again. What shame! I had turned into a virtual recluse. I avoided the day and only sneaked out at night whenever necessary. I tried to minimize my leakage. Since I discovered that the less I ate or drank, the less stool and urine leaked out, I resorted to having only one meal a day, with minimal or no fluids at all.

I did this mostly for my husband. However, when my weight took a dive due to under-eating, it alienated him even more. At times, when he was around and I joined him in bed, he would find an excuse to walk out. My friends were no longer visiting due to my delicate state. Several times, feeling helpless, alone and betrayed, I would entertain the thought of overdosing myself with a mixture of drugs to death – which I did. But death too did not want me, it ran away from me.

One afternoon when Mark was away, like most other days, I swallowed a mixture of antibiotics, painkillers and other medicines that I could find. I did not have a proper understanding of what drugs could induce death, but I imagined that if I took all the drugs that I could lay my hands on at the same time, there was no possible way I would remain alive. I had left Mark a letter on the bed, stating that I loved him and I was responsible for the loss of his child. But I did not die. I only earned myself a terrible stomachache and a migraine.

Months on end, Mark's coldness grew worse. He no longer ate the food I prepared for him. I would serve him food and he would claim to be full or he lacked appetite. Two weeks before he suggested I head to his parents, he reinvigorated his warmth towards me. He was no longer condescending or cold. Sometimes he would help me with the house chores. I was happy that his anger had finally gone down and he was now at peace with the death and with me. I was elated that he had promised to get me help regarding my situation. When he finally asked me to go live with his parents, he guaranteed me comfort and adequate care by his folks.

Three weeks had elapsed already. Mark had neither come to visit nor called even once. His number was equally off.

"Why did you get married to our son?" Mark's mother would ask every time she felt like it.

The question assumed a rhetoric undertone. She did not want an answer. She wanted me to leave her son, yet she could not say it directly. Just like Mark, they were bitter about the dead child, silently placing the blame on me. They were also disgusted by my condition, which they could not find a solution to, as my husband had assured me. Most of the people around the home thought I was possessed, if not the devil itself. They avoided me like a plague.

I was worried about Mark when the fourth week rolled in without a word from him. I was also overwhelmed by my unappreciated stay at his parents' place. Since he was not coming to me, I took the wise step to go to him. Perhaps he was sick, or had been robbed or something terrible that I did not want to imagine had happened to him. I was careful to wear lots of underclothing and avoided eating and drinking in an effort to avoid the travelling humiliation that befell me earlier.

It was almost 6 p.m. when I arrived in Kisumu city where he lived. I was anxious to see my husband. Normally, he got home from work at five, so I was sure to find him. I was already prepared to understand why he could not manage to visit or send a message. At times, he could get very busy and I understood this. My shock would however be overwhelming. Mark no longer resided in the house we used to.

"He moved a month ago," one of the neighbours announced.

I was devastated. I felt crushed. I was bitter. I felt betrayed again. While I innocently went to the village, he had packed and moved houses that very day. Nobody knew where he had moved to. Milkah, one of our old neighbours, allowed me stay at her place for the night and until I picked myself up. However, my stay was short-lived. She kicked me out the following day after wetting her bed.

I decided to go back to Mark's parents' home in Homa Bay. As an orphan, I had nowhere else to go anyway.

When I arrived at the home, I could hear sounds of jubilation from a distance. I did not immediately decipher what was going on. There were plenty of songs in the air, and clearly, I could tell that they were coming from Mark's home. When I inched closer and the sounds began assuming human shapes and motion, I correctly concluded that in fact, the songs and jubilation were accompanied by dancing.

I moved closer. Mark's face and mine met. It was clear – I was an unwanted visitor! Next to him was a pompous young girl. They were both dressed in matching *vitenge* suits, symbolic of love and unity. Mark's father stood behind the two with a huge smile plastered on his face. He held in his hands a traditional whisk, the kind that custom only allows you to hold when you are blessing your son for marriage, and Mark's father was a man of customs.

At that moment, I knew that it was over between us. I felt dizzy. I wanted to throw up but the urge just melted away. I recollected myself and walked to the bus stop alone, in silence. I had no idea where to go or whom to call for help. But as fate would have it, a woman from the local church saw me cry; she thought I was bereaved! She took me into her house where I stayed for a week incognito. It was during this time that my friend Janet brought good news from the church. She said that there was a church notice about a free camp to help women leaking urine after childbirth to be held in the county referral hospital. How would I get there? I wondered. Little did I know that Janet had spoken to the priest who would facilitate my transport to this hospital. Here, at least women leaking urine like me were dignified.

It has been a week since my operation. It is indeed unbelievable that I leak no more! Although I do not know where to go after discharge, the most important thing for me is that I am not leaking any more. It is the best thing that has happened to me in a long time! These days I sleep like a baby – no leakage *manenos* and no worries. I cannot ask for more. May God favour the staff at the hospital that treated me, who endured the smell and the mess in their line of duty. This is indeed a calling and not just a duty.

Out of Turn

When the doctors decided that what was ailing me was something they called Vesico-Vaginal Fistula (VVF), I did not have the slightest idea how different my life was going to be, beginning that moment. As a community darling, the greatest dancer to ever have been born in Visanga village, at the very least, I expected bags of sympathy and a public display of solidarity. I had lived for the public, I belonged to the public, I entertained them, turned their sad days into sunshine and now I was walking back to them expecting to receive only half of what I had given them. Sitting in that vehicle from Visanga District Hospital, I determined that my first stop would be the marketplace where I had lived all my life.

The minibus arrived at Visanga Market just as the market women were locking up their stalls to wind up for the day. Quietly with the aid of darkness, I slipped through the crowds of people, my head bent and covered by a turban, and headed straight to the back corridor leading to my boyfriend's shop. I did not intend to waste any time: I had to confront him.

I bought some time walking aimlessly around the shop until the last customer left. He was closing the front door to the shop when I got to where he was.

"You should have told me I was giving my body to a boy who has no capacity to man up," I challenged him, clapping my hands sarcastically. I could see that when Kegora turned, he was both surprised to see me and agitated by my choice of words.

"Don't talk to me like that young girl. What are you doing here?" he shot back.

"You ripped my body apart and now I have brought it back to you to repair it or marry it," I hissed.

"Woman, stop shouting! I have had a long day at work and the last thing I need is a woman bickering around my ears. Get out of here!" That, I was certain, was an order, dispatched in a tone that I was familiar with – the tone that was often followed by clenched fists and a typical display of violence as was common with any cornered man in our community. However, I was not prepared to stop speaking.

"If you are man enough," I shouted even louder, "… then show me where our child is buried!"

My case was simple. Kegora impregnated me and left me to my own means: he never bothered to know what I would eat during my pregnancy, where I would sleep, how I would get to hospital, what would become of our child, let alone attempt to find out the gender of the child. Then after nine months of pregnancy, three days of labour and an hour of surgery, the doctor removed from my womb a dead child, whose legacy was what the doctor called Vesico-Vaginal Fistula.

Yes, I was angry, and perhaps that anger was what precluded me from having clarity, or rather the simple memory of how easily agitated Kegora's masculinity was under this kind of circumstance, where I took him head-on in an argument. I think the weight which the blow he landed on me carried was heavily influenced by the expectations he felt he had to meet of the small crowd that had begun gathering. I had asked for it and now I was on the floor writhing in pain.

I fell right on the urine bag of the catheter which burst open, spewing a bit of waste on some of the faces that were cheering the drama. Other parts of the catheter disintegrated, with my skirt taking a journey far above where it was supposed to be, leaving my body exposed. The silence that followed was palpable. The cheers quickly disappeared and the silence was only broken by a loud voice calling me a witch.

"Witch! Witch! Witch! Witch!" Several voices picked up the branding, which grew into a chant as they edged closer to me.

The suggestion of witchcraft seemed to emanate from the installation of foreign objects on my body which they, just like me a few days ago, did not know what they were. To make matters worse, a courageous member of the crowd grabbed the urine bag, smelt it and identified the content to be urine, which he said was in fact the most concentrated urine he had ever encountered in his entire life. There was no time to wonder if he went around smelling people's urine, given that my life was on the cliff at that moment.

Witchcraft in our community was a diverse constituency, but among the most commonly-shared understanding was the idea that to bewitch somebody, you needed at least something that was known to be in contact with the human body. A witch would ask you to bring hair strands, saliva of the person you wanted to cast a spell on, a pint of blood, someone's sweat, garment or even, as was conceived in this case, urine. Strangely enough, while witches were widely accepted as a part of the community, they thrived in secrecy. Once you were known to have sought the services of one, you had to pay a price and the price for witchcraft was death by stoning.

"It's not what you think …," I attempted to defend myself as the crowd charged towards me.

"… Hospital … I am from hospital …," I continued to plead. They became deaf.

"Please … please! Let me explain!" They still kept charging towards me.

I looked around to spot Kegora for help. I could not see him.

"Bring a car tyre!" shouted one person.

"Burn her! Burn her …," more chants picked up.

I could have been roasted alive. Except that my stomach had refused to deflate after I had given birth. Having pleaded with all the words I could grasp, what saved me in the end was the shrill persistent voice of a woman who formed a song out of the words, "That woman is pregnant, leave her alone!"

Pregnancy, even when imagined, has a way of speaking to the soul of every man and woman. By the time the crowd hesitantly dispersed, I was scared to my last breath. The woman who had saved me was all there was left around me, accompanied by darkness, a galaxy of stars in the sky and the ominous hooting of a disappointed owl. Owls could kill to see death, we believed.

"What do you think you are doing, showing your body to people?" the woman blurted out.

"Showing what?" I asked, genuinely confused and still in deep pain.

"The catheter. You foolish woman, that is our secret!"

Sarah, as I learnt was her name, held my hand and supported me back to my feet. In silence and darkness, she walked me through the deserted market, past a few closed shops and finally to the doorstep of a *posho* mill. She reached into her pouch, fished out a bunch of keys and struggled to find the one that opened our pathway into the *posho* mill.

There was a mattress on the floor just next to the grinding machine. "I live here," she said, almost in a whisper.

Sarah prepared kales, which we ate with *ugali* after she showed me where to clean myself up. It was literally outside where darkness provided me the cover that ordinarily the four walls of a bathroom would. She also gave me her clothes and some leftover diapers, which we confirmed had long exhausted the gap between the date of manufacture and the expiry date. Finally, we settled down to talk, one on one, after I recovered from the shock.

"I have mine too," she told me with a smile while pulling up her dress, as I spread a shawl on the floor and sat with my back against the wall. I could see that she had her catheter *in situ*. For a moment I did not know what crossed my mind, but in my heart, the feeling I had was that of comradeship.

"You too …?" I asked, suddenly returning to reality.

"Yes," she said. It shocked me when she further revealed that it was her seventeenth year battling fistula. "I was fourteen when I became expectant," she disclosed. Her family history with pregnancy, just like mine, involved traditional midwives. On the second day of her labour when it was clear that the midwives had exhausted their knowledge on what to do, a quick decision was arrived at to send Sarah to hospital. Nevertheless, her pregnancy had its own plans and halfway through the journey to the hospital aboard a wheelbarrow, the foetus demanded to be born urgently. She pushed it out and for a minute, Sarah had the chance of holding her baby before the child breathed its last within the first hour of living. The child simply gave up in life.

"The chap was born in the wrong world," Sarah jibed, referring to her dead child. "He noticed it soon enough … brilliant fellow … and decided to check out without wasting much time."

Despite the joke in her choice of words, I could see her eyes becoming wet and shiny. I wiped her tears with my hand. From the day of her child's birth, she carried the trauma of losing a child and the consequences of being handled by midwives, whose experience was limited to less complex pregnancies and who clearly were out of turn for the case Sarah presented to them. They, according to information Sarah later received from a medic, did not do a good job of stitching her up. They cut her up to fulfil what was required during the second stage of labour where the opening for the baby to pass through needed to be quickly enlarged, except that the cutting happened on both sides. The doctors called this *bilateral episiotomy*, which was worsened by the child making a further tearing, hence opening the pathway for the fistula.

I was sorry for her, forgetting my own situation temporarily. Never had I seen a woman with the fistula problem in my community. The first time I heard of the condition was the day my prognosis was made.

Ordinarily, it was not easy to really tell if someone had a fistula because this was a shameful condition, I learnt.

"How come I have never seen you in this community?" I finally found the space to ask her what was on my mind.

She laughed briefly then told me, "I have seen you. You dance every Friday at the market dais. You dance beautifully, but you know that has to stop now."

"I don't get it…"

"You will… you sure will."

She stood up. "I have to empty this," she said, pointing to her urine bag. I also took the chance to go and relieve myself.

"Do you go to church?" she asked when we both came back into the room.

"Yes… why?" I asked

"Forget about going to church again."

"I dance in the choir."

"Not anymore. No more dancing."

"Why?"

She took a long pause, then rose to add some more food to her plate.

"You said you have never seen me…" I was not sure if that was a question, but I nodded my head affirmatively anyway. "You have earned your ticket to take a turn out of sight."

"I don't understand you," I genuinely said.

"You will!" she affirmed.

I felt for some reason that moment reminded me of the heaviness in my mind. When a few hours before I looked up for Kegora's help and he was out of sight, it occurred to me that once again, he had slipped out of my life, just as my parents and his parents had. Unsolicited pregnancy, as my father called it, had made me a pariah at home, at only seventeen years old. My stay in my father's compound had concluded for now. As he had observed, I had decided to prove myself woman enough and therefore I should immediately have depended upon myself and the facilitator of my pregnancy to set up a home of my own, which he determined would even be easier for me given that out of 'compassion', he had written off my dowry. Now without that very child who determined my pathway, without that man who treated me as a chameleon would, without that confidence to dance on the dais again and without a clue of what lay ahead, I had only that night to think about the rest of my life – whether it would be that night alone or the next many years. I just did not know.

Surgical experiences

Background

While surgery plays a significant role in correcting fistula cases, it also poses a lot of challenges. This is mainly because only a few facilities where surgical repair services can be undertaken are available; a situation that is made worse by the low number of specialists available to carry out the procedure. This, pitted against the wide spread of the problem in Africa. Another fundamental challenge that arises is the lack of a proper referral mechanism that interlinks communication between one hospital and another, where when a patient is referred for treatment to another hospital, the secondary hospital is not aware of the case. This delays the pace at which emergencies can be handled and further takes out from the equation a progress report that may be shared between the handlers of the affected women. The stories in this section look at how entrenched this problem is.

Veiled Bliss

I resisted him despite his kindness. He did not understand. Who in their right mind would want to marry a woman who could not control her stool and urine from leaking? He must have been a fool. 'Jacob is indeed a fool', I thought to myself. When everybody was running away from me because I smelt like manure and sewage, Jacob was embracing me and cleaning my mess. What drove him? I would look at him in my silent moments and laugh and wonder.

"I love and adore you Doreen," Jacob would say, and the statement would throw me into bouts of wild laughter.

'This one does not know the monster that fistula is,' I would say to myself and laugh again.

I had nursed too much suffering to pity myself anymore. I had been betrayed. I had been abused. I had been chased away and treated like a pariah. I imagined that when Jacob would get tired of my leakages and the humiliation I would bring into his life by my fistula, his next move would not catch me by surprise. It was a predictable pattern that had happened many times over. My conscience had built an immunity around rejection and betrayal. With a smile and a thankful tongue, I would walk out of his house with my fistula and wait for my death, which was hesitating to meet me in spite of the many unsuccessful attempts.

However, Jacob's 'madness' seemed to be growing by the day. He was now proposing that I should accompany him to church. "God will make a way," he would say.

"Which God? There is no God, Jacob," I would shoot back. "There is only suffering, pain and death."

"Doreen, I have seen the hand of God…"

"Ahaa! Where has that hand been when my family abandoned me, when I lost my job, when I leaked urine like a child? Is God aware that people call me the mighty urine sprinkler, the cursed one? There is no God!" I would stamp with finality.

The idea of God irritated me. It angered me. But Jacob would not tire of telling me that he had prayed for me to see that very hand of God that he too had seen. Whenever his church members would gather in our little home to pray for me, I would sneak out while their eyes remained closed, calling on their nonexistent God. Yet, they would never hold their noses or talk behind my back like everyone else. Were their noses blocked? Were they blind in the few instances urine would drip in their presence? Ironically, they would thank God because of me. Believers are peculiar people.

It was a Tuesday evening. Jacob was back home when I walked into the house. He was dancing as he loved to do. He was not a very good dancer. It was embarrassing to watch, but I reserved my comments and endured the unfortunate scene.

"We made it, praise God, we made it," Jacob sang, slowing on his dance.

"Made what … were we making anything?" I asked anxiously.

"Surgery, your money for a fistula surgery darling," he replied enthusiastically.

I was dumbfounded and confused for a while. Confused too. We had not been looking for any funds. Furthermore, the cost of surgery was way beyond Jacob's little pay. What was he talking about? It was not a funny joke in case he was trying to pull my leg. Despite my immunity to ridicule and abuse regarding my condition, that had crossed the line.

It hit me like a thunderbolt of shock and guilt. Could mankind go to that extent? So much inhumane treatment can make one fear or laugh away any kind act. I had rejected them with their God. I had laughed at their efforts to intercede my case with God. My unbelief and disregard of them did not ruffle their efforts to find a solution to my long suffering. They would go on, silently organizing fundraisers, unbeknownst to me. I was overwhelmed by a nameless emotion. I was afraid to look at them when they came over to officially extend warm wishes and prayers for a successful surgery. My heart was heavy, my lips were sealed, numbed too, and I could not find words to apologize, to thank them. With their sharp powers of intuition, they would read the guilt masking my face, my helplessness, and shoot a comforting smile at me.

"It shall be well; we thank the Almighty," they chorused.

Fear gripped me. My anxiety levels had hit the roof. What if it failed?

The thought of a medical accident flooded my mind. The pain might be unbearable. I could not endure the graphic images of shining scalpels tearing through my flesh like a piece of paper. "You shall be fine," Jacob comfortingly whispered. We quietly marched into the hospital to be booked in for the operation.

I was shown into what they called a holding area. Each step I made into it severed a nerve in me. The hospital environment was not one I would ever reconcile with. To me, the hospital represented a dark image: where my brother lost his leg to amputation; where my grandmother was confined for six months ravaged by the cruelty of cancer. She was in pain. Unimaginable suffering. The hospital was a constant and disturbing memory of my own child that I never got to see smile. It housed all the ugly images of humanity's sufferings. I hated it. The smell of antiseptic, medicine and sickness gave me an olfactory fatigue. The uniformed men and women marching in and out of rooms to inflict pain on innocent sufferers with their syringes scared me. Did they have to inflict pain to relieve pain?

"Hello, how are you today? I am Caren…," a middle-aged lady attired in blue walked into the room, greeting me and smiling youthfully. "I am your operating nurse and I shall be part of the operating team," she added.

Would a nurse smiling that youthfully be able to battle my twelve-year experience with fistula? I doubted it. She did not have the rough and serious face that could scare away a virus or a disease.

"What is your name and your date of birth?" she asked while maintaining her smile, exposing her spotless white teeth.

"Doreen … Doreen Moraa," I stammered.

She took down the details while still smiling. I failed to conceive her source of persistent joy. What was her problem, smiling all the time?

"What is the name of your surgeon?" she continued.

I did not understand her question. Why was she asking me about things that they already knew? Or did they imagine that I carried my own surgeon along?

Earlier on, I had met a team of jovial men and women cloaked in blue attire. They introduced themselves as the team that would be operating on me. I was initially afraid. Why so many people? I had thought that my problem was not too big to be handled by such a group. They had to assemble an entire hospital team to handle me! This reignited my fear. Perhaps I would never heal. Perhaps I would not come out alive. I was terribly afraid. Although their smiles and jocular nature were meant to calm me, they did not. One could never be calm when death or pain was imminent. I was more terrified when she asked me what surgery I would be having. I was not a surgeon myself. *Isn't it the work of the surgeons to know more, and to know better?* I thought.

As soon as she was out, an old fellow with a brown moustache walked in and introduced himself as the anesthesiologist – the one in charge of putting me in a half-dead state. The way he spoke truly reflected his professional skills of putting operation candidates into an unconscious state. He talked musically, his inflections and tone in control, perhaps deliberately to calm me. Jack assured me of maximum comfort before, during and after the operation. I almost protested that I did not want comfort; it was not what took me there – fistula did. Their individual continuous flow in and out of the room heightened my anxiety. The process was becoming more like an election exercise.

As I was wheeled into the operating room dressed in a blue gown, I felt as though I was being marched to my grave alive. The sight of the armoury of operation tools made my heart race. It was disturbing to imagine that all those weapons were meant to invade my body to fight the stubborn fistula. I was not ready. As I slid from the stretcher to the operating bed, I lied that I wanted to use the washrooms. Caren offered to show me around but unbeknownst to her, I was not planning to come back to the operating room. It was too terrifying. I would rather have suffered the leakages that I was used to, than risk death by a process fraught with fear and anxiety and without a comprehensive guarantee that it would heal me.

Paralysed by the fear and unfounded confusion, I bolted from the washrooms in my theatre gown to the direction I thought would lead me out of that house of pain and death. But my failed attempted escape from the scalpels only earned me more hours of counselling sessions to convince me of the seamless process that would happen while I was unconscious.

At my second wheeling into the operating room, there was a sudden downpour and wild thunder and lightning. That was not a good sign, I told them. We grew up fanning the belief that lightning was a symbol of bad luck since it signalled an end to the rains, which were a symbol of blessings. I again declined to be wheeled into the theatre. The wild storms evoked all of the horrific images and tales buried in my subconscious, further deepening my fear. The team of surgeons, ironically, did not seem irritated. They observed me patiently with their trained professional glances punctuated with smiles and understanding. They were determined that nothing would injure their joy of service, borne out of the long years of patience and pain in surgery classes. Just like the believers, nothing fazed them, they had a permanent resolve to attain their ends.

I was back to that very bed, the one that would witness the battle between fistula and the battalion of surgeons. An unusually cold temperature dominated the operating room alongside the flurry of activities. I walked my eyes from nurse to nurse, each putting up the surgical ensemble, working in perfect harmony and in militarized organization. On the right side, a monitor displayed my blood pressure readings, my breathing and my heart rate. A tight wrapper passed from one side of the bed, across my thighs to the other side of the bed. I imagined that they thought I would bolt again never to reappear. Caren, the operating nurse, was back beside the bed smiling and armed with petty records.

"What is your name and date of birth?"

"What surgery are you having?" she inquired again.

I asked them whether they had misplaced my details, or if I had been mistaken for someone else. I remembered the anecdote of the man who could not distinguish between circumcision and castration and ended up undergoing the latter instead of the former. I was scared that they would mix up my innocent body parts and operate on the wrong ones.

"Normal verification procedure," the three nurses sang in unison.

I do not remember how I drifted into unconsciousness. Nobody knows the exact time or minute they fall asleep. The only memory I have, a blurred memory, is Caren's beautiful smile as she spoke to the surgeon.

"Done!" she said.

After what must have been endless hours away from earth, I began to hear fuzzy voices, which went on for some time until I popped my eyes open.

"Congratulations!" a familiar voice said. I struggled to wipe away the confusion in my eyes. I was almost startled out of bed. "You did it."

"Did what?" I inquired as I fully regained my senses. Caren watched me with the brilliance of her smile, her hands gently pushing the stretcher that would introduce me to the recovery room. I had one question to ask the nurses, the one that mattered the most.

"Does this mean that I am well? No more leakages?" I inquired with an anxious face. Caren smiled and softly gripped my shoulders.

Just then, I thought of Jacob – his unimaginable love and the sacrifices the church members had made to ensure that the surgery took place. A deep feeling of indebtedness overwhelmed me I was wheeled past the sterile corridor walls of the hospital. I could not wait to meet and embrace him.

One More Attempt

Down Shelly Beach, South Coast of Mombasa, Kenya, the ocean breeze sweeps past the sandy beach into the quiet of the town. It was an ordinary Sunday morning except for Milka and her husband Justus, lying on the cabana beds spread across the ocean line, mostly frequented by tourists. Milka was about to make a milestone in her twenty-five-year fistula journey and for her, there was no better place for that than the ocean-side.

The two of them, husband and wife, had not had the best moments together recently. Milka felt that Justus had lived through the past years disliking her, and she coped through that imagined dislike with a plateful of indifference. The friction between them was visible. It was the first time they were out together for luxury, just the two of them.

"I hope you are not planning to swim in the ocean," Justus mumbled to Milka with a concerned tone.

"Why?" Milka asked.

"You need to take a shower first if you want to swim," Justus responded, unaware of the weight of his words.

Milka did not want to waste time. She was already too fed up with him to bother and after that comment, she figured it was the best time to table her thoughts.

"I am leaving you Justus," she said.

A minute passed in silence. Two kids were playing at the beach, splashing sand at each other and laughing rowdily. Their excitement only served to elevate the juxtaposition which was completed by the silence on the cabana beds.

Justus did not utter a word. He stood up, took a walk towards the foot of the ocean and stood gazing at the water mass.

Milka joined him.

"You need a better woman, someone that can satisfy you," she said to him.

"Where is this coming from Milka? What wrong have I done?" Justus faced her. He looked prepared for a confrontation.

"It's not you. It's me," she said.

"Fistula?"

"Yes."

For eighteen years, they lived together aware of the fistula and gave each other a shoulder to lean on. The last three years however, after her fourth failed surgery, had been tumultuous. Milka simply gave up, and that was where the problem began. She gave up on herself and on the prospects of a future together.

In fact, after insistence from Justus, the two had only managed to go to a hospital twice since the surgery three years before. The last visit included spending a huge sum of money paid to a private practitioner who gave Milka some six nondescript and expensive tablets to insert in her vagina every night for seven days and thirty other tablets to swallow each night. When they failed to make any impact, all hope was lost for Milka.

In Mikindani, Mombasa where the two lived, poverty was rampant. People had no money; many families experienced hunger, making home delivery the better option for many pregnant women. At the time of her disastrous pregnancy twenty-five years before, she, like many women in her community, had no chance of accessing proper healthcare. Her option of giving birth at home suffered a series of complications, which eventually led her to giving birth on the way to hospital. The baby weighed 3.6 kgs and died two hours after birth – after enduring labour for almost three days. Three days after the infant's death, she noticed her bedding becoming wet one day after another. At the time, she had no idea she had developed a fistula, having never experienced anything like that before or seen any woman with such a problem.

For her to live through the problem for twenty-five years, she could not perceive any other way that the issue could be resolved. She was not one of those women who believed that they were cursed or carried some kind of generational hoodoo; in fact, she took every chance she got with the possibility of medical intervention. She believed in science, science which had failed her.

Things went downhill from that point. She took less care of herself, showered less frequently and was not bothered by what society said about her. She lost it!

If there was someone who suffered the consequences of her decisions first-hand, it had to be Justus. In two weeks, he fled from the master bedroom which had turned into a toilet.

Luckily, their daughter Faith, now twenty-one, was away from home, studying at the university. Many of the problems they faced were between them, given that Milka rarely stepped outside the house. She had given up on society too.

"Look at me and tell me I have not done everything possible to care for you, to be there for you?" Justus asked Milka in a resigned voice.

"You are too good for me, that is why I have to leave," Milka said. Her tone was sincere, but if you were on the other side, on Justus's side, all you saw was ungratefulness, arrogance and condescension.

"I don't deserve you; don't you get it?" she screamed.

The two kids who were playing by the beach got caught up in the drama, unbeknown to Milka and Justus.

"I get it! I get it!" shouted the two children simultaneously, involving themselves in the adult conversation jokingly and having fun while at it. Justus descended on them with slaps, measured to fit what a father would give to his own children in respect of the biblical instruction – spare the rod and spoil the child.

"Get away from here you two brats!" he yelled at them. Clearly you could tell that the anger he exuded had its origin elsewhere.

When Faith, their daughter, turned eighteen, Milka had felt a responsibility to induct her into what motherhood could become. It was the first time she revealed to her daughter that she suffered from fistula, bringing the total number of persons aware of her condition within the family and community to three: Justus, herself and now her daughter.

It was a consensus-based decision to tell Faith. She, they concluded, had become a big girl and anything happening to her mother, she should know. Telling her helped in many ways. She became part of the fistula care process for the mother, sometimes even helping her to clean the rags she used as sanitary pads and air them on the drying line, encouraging her and even reminding her to take her medication.

In her community, Milka believed she was the only one with the fistula problem. After all, it is not easy to really tell who had a fistula because it was a shameful condition. People did not talk about it openly and in any case, what was the point of telling, yet one would not receive any help from anywhere? It was pointless.

Her last visit to the hospital was what introduced her to the second woman she would know to have fistula in the village. It was this visit that put her on the path to desiring a divorce. The woman had lived with her husband for 14 years with no child. Both the husband and wife were very resilient about it. That was until in the fifteenth year, the husband brought home another wife, sending her to Siberia. Milka had never imagined that one day she would be separated from her husband, but not after hearing that confession. She was convinced that it was a matter of when, not if. She had to leave before she was left.

"Really Milka? Is that what you really believe?" Justus reacted with a sarcastic laugh. He had prodded her to explain herself, particularly why she wanted to abandon a marriage of more than a quarter of a century. That was the story she told him.

"If that woman could be left by her husband, what stops you from leaving me?" Milka asked him.

"I am not that woman's husband. Not all men are the same."

"Isn't that what all men say?"

"So now you are in touch with all men to know what they say?"

There was silence again. It dawned on Justus that what his wife needed was not divorce, but reassurance.

"I will allow you to leave me," Justus said, "but only if you do for me one last thing."

"What?"

Something different filled the air. It was possible that in bringing up the idea of divorce, Milka had hoped it would not remain on the table, yet now it seemed to scare her that it was actually being considered. She feared for what the condition could be.

"We give surgery one more chance. If it succeeds, leave me. If it fails, stay with me until it is successful. Can you do that for me?"

He had edged closing to her, closing the gap between them and they could feel each other's breath.

"Yes, I can," Milka responded.

She was subdued by the heavy presence of her husband's manliness, which had dominated the environment. "Although I am an adult learner in an evening school, I have not disclosed this to the teacher. He keeps sending me messages to find out why I dropped out when

I should be joining secondary school, but I have not disclosed this to him either."

Three weeks later, the two of them, now joined by Faith, held hands at the national referral hospital.

"All indications point to the surgery being successful," said the doctor, towering over them. Faith jumped up, celebrating.

"Don't celebrate yet; it's too early. We have to monitor progress before we arrive at any conclusion," the doctor advised.

He handed Justus a small handbook and sent Faith to find a specific nurse from the lobby. The nurse was inexistent, a clever way for the hospital staff to keep the children far enough for long enough and give the adults a chance to talk.

"Now that the surgery is done, how long should we abstain from sexual intercourse?" Justus asked. Milka expressed surprise.

"Six months. But it is also advisable to ensure that you have a reliable family planning method to prevent pregnancy for at least two years. Next time you get pregnant, remember to inform your healthcare provider about your fistula history. The information will be very important in planning appropriate care for you and your baby," the doctor replied.

Milka smiled. "I will add a bonus of two months, giving myself a total of eight months of abstinence," she said. Everyone laughed.

"No more babies coming soon, maybe in ten years," Justus added.

During Faith's graduation, precisely three years after that day, Milka and Justus walked to the graduation square holding hands. The graduation party ended late in the day and they could not find a place to sleep. All hotels around were booked. They found themselves in the outskirts of town in a dingy place that looked like it alternated between hosting humans and animals.

"I can't believe this is where we will sleep," Milka said.

"Do you remember the way you suffered, sleeping on a plastic paper? Getting wet all night long?" Justus joked.

"It's all in the past," she said, smiling.

Dingy as the place was, something came out of it. Faith had finished school, they were lonely and growing old. They needed company, and what better time to get company than when they were far from their past, far from home and far from the recommended two years a fistula survivor should wait until the next pregnancy?

Confluence

When you are fourteen years old and pregnant, your options in life suffer a fatal blow. The first blow for me was my boyfriend, sixteen-year-old Richard who was a class ahead of me, looking me straight in the eye and advising me to erase every memory we had shared together.

"Martha, we only slept together once, how can you be pregnant?" he shot at me.

"I am pregnant, I am telling you the truth," I pleaded with him.

"I am not even old enough to impregnate a girl who herself is not old enough to be pregnant," he defended himself.

Richard was the son of the school headteacher and we both understood that this was not the kind of news you happily walked into the headteacher's office with. We were cooked, and we knew it!

"Have you ever told your parents that we slept together?" Richard asked me.

"How could I?" What kind of a question was that?

"How about your friends?"

"No!"

"Have you ever told anyone?"

"No!"

"Then you and I are done. We do not know each other and nothing has ever transpired between us. I hope that is clear enough." With that, Richard walked away. He never stopped to say hallo to me or even acknowledge my presence any time we met after that day. Two weeks later, when my morning sickness ratted me out, his father took a stroll with me to the school gate and told me, "Now Martha, follow this road. It will take you to the market centre where your fellow mothers are. The only time I expect to see you in this school again is when you are bringing your child to join us."

I had survived beatings from the headteacher, but as they say, your lucky stars shine only once. Starting from that day and for the next eight months, my mother kept confusing me with a punching bag. Anything that went wrong in her house was associated with me. I became the senseless girl whose priority in life was to be foolish and even if a glass broke or something else went amiss, it certainly had to be the senseless girl who was not clever enough to keep things together.

"If she can break her virginity at fourteen, what stops her from breaking a mere glass?" my mother once quipped.

It was after one of those turbulent days when the worst happened. I was inching closer to what was supposed to be my due date. As usual, something went amiss in the house and I immediately assumed my position as the usual suspect. A kick from my mother must have missed the target I suppose, because up to this day, I am not convinced that my stomach was the intended target. I fell flat on the floor and lay flat on the hospital bed for the next six months. Needless to say, I lost my child in the process.

My pregnancy had been kept a secret, hidden even from my older sisters who were happily married. I remember that after losing my child, it became apparent to everyone that I had failed to tow the moral line. At one point, one of my elder sisters paid me a visit at the hospital.

"Is this Martha at the age of fourteen?" she asked rhetorically.

"I sent her to school to open books, but she went ahead to open her legs for men instead," my mother, who was present, responded. It was not that part of the response that bothered me; I was used to it. It was what she said after.

"She could not put brakes on her nether region, now the very region has lost all brakes. She has developed a fistula as a bonus to her failed pregnancy," my mother added. I did not understand what a fistula was, but soon enough I did. I realized that some of the bottles hanging around my hospital bed were not necessarily 'drips' for intravenous fluids. I became familiar with the language of catheters.

That day was the last day anyone came visiting for the six months I was there. I had also developed nerve damage on my left leg, which was part of the reasons my stay was extended. When I started to walk a bit, one sympathetic nurse whom I had grown fond of organized for my escape from the hospital, given that it was impossible that I would ever be able to settle the hospital bill which had accumulated.

Upon my escape, I reasoned against going home; instead, I chose to go stay with my other sister who lived near Kisii Town. I lived with my sister for some time. She was not very comfortable with me either; she would talk about me with her neighbours.

One day I sat at the dinner table with my sister, her husband and her two children. Her husband was a biology teacher at one of the top schools in the region, a quiet man who talked only if he had to. He suggested, "I think we can put some money together and take Martha to hospital for surgery at the end of this month."

There was an immediate uproar.

"Our money! Never! I would rather use that money as tissue paper than take her to hospital," my sister sneered and cut him short. That was the end of that discussion. I had previously argued with her during the day over a different matter and I therefore assumed that she was displacing her anger over the previous argument. But again, I thought to myself that if she could say that, then what was in her mind was not too far from what she said.

My sister once told a neighbour that she had developed a skin rash because I used her washing basin. They talked about me all the time. She even went as far as telling our relatives not to visit because I smelt. There was very little I could do because after all, my own mother had forsaken me. I felt useless. I cried a lot. I had nowhere to hide, no one to comfort me. I was all alone in the midst of this situation. Many times, I contemplated suicide.

One time, I reached my breaking point and went to buy rat poison. This, as suggested to me by my childhood stories, was said to have the capacity to end human life. On my way back from the agrovet, I bumped into a friend, Gertrude, who worked as a house-help for one of the townspeople. My unsettledness gave me away and I found myself giving an account of my life to her in that short moment.

"The way you smile at people, how could we tell you were a full movie of problems?" Gertrude joked. For some reason, perhaps due to the tone she used, we laughed. I had not had a good laugh in a long time, but that day a few minutes to what was supposed to be the end of me, I laughed and laughed hard.

"I know someone who can help you," she told me.

"Help me? With my leakage?" I asked, surprised.

"Do I look like a magician? Your leakage is your problem, but the bigger problem you have is that you need a job. Then you can afford treatment."

A week after that conversation, I stole just enough money for my transport from my sister's handbag and fled off in the dead of the night to Nairobi, Kenya's capital city and land of opportunities.

My first job as a house-help was at a home where Gertrude had worked before returning back to Kisii at her husband's behest. Sadly, I only managed to work in this new home for three days.

"We cannot stretch our stay with you any further," was my dismissal notice. I was paid a full month's salary and released in good faith the next day. The salary gave me a starting point and allowed me movement as I searched for my next landing place. I found my way.

For three years during this time when I was working as a house-help, I changed jobs as soon as the bosses started complaining about a funny smell in their house. Others would discharge me in a polite way saying, "Take three months' leave, we will call you back."

I did not disclose to any of them what was wrong with me. They would not understand, I was convinced. I lived my life the best way I could. At one time, I worked for my cousin for one whole year without pay. Finally, they threw me out like a dog on the ground that my interaction with the bathroom needed a review, which they lacked the necessary qualifications to assist me with. That was when I made the decision to go back to Kisii Town. This was perhaps my most timely decision ever.

"Hi," my seatmate in the Kisii-bound bus greeted me.

"Hi," I smiled back.

Two months later, on the banks of River Mogonga, which flows into Lake Victoria, the man I had met on the bus, Ogembo, looked into my eyes and asked me to be his girlfriend. By this time, I was living with my other cousin and Ogembo and I had visited each other quite frequently. He had come to know of my condition, which was the first thing I told him when I started to notice signs of a man falling in love.

"We will find some money and get you treated," he said.

Ogembo was no angel, but he was all I ever wanted. He was a teacher and was more familiar with fistula as a societal issue than me who lived with it. He was also a divorcé who, in his words, had married a Westernized woman that could not accommodate the needs of an African man. He ran away from the marriage as soon as he realized that even after paying dowry, his wife still demanded equality in the house. Cooking, washing clothes and utensils, babysitting and all other feminine responsibilities were now to be divided right down the middle.

"She had the audacity of imbibing alcohol in my presence; which woman does that?" Ogembo presented the situation to me. He was a traditional man and to that extent, I understood him. Personally, while I held a separate opinion, having lived with many modernized families in the city, my background as a house-help made house chores easy for me and I viewed it more as a duty than a burden. I actually loved to put things in order.

With Ogembo, we survived many wars. Villagers invented one name after another and slung them my way, and sometimes our way. They called us *amache esosera* (stagnant rainwater) or *mobochoku*! (the hollow one). The name-calling would come in different contextual forms, for example, "*Amache esosera* (stagnant rainwater) is passing by".

Ogembo had accepted me in spite of the fistula. He slept with me in the same bed and bought all my sanitary towels when my own family never wanted to see me. I knew that any hope I had of ever repaying his kindness was pegged on surgery. It was all we talked about whenever the social pressure rose.

After months of saving, we had finally arrived at a reasonable figure for the surgery.

We packed our bags, ready to travel to Nairobi. In the morning as we left the house hand in hand, it occurred to us that we could benefit from the counsel of a doctor at the local general hospital who had been a pillar in our lives. The hospital, we determined, would be our first stop since we had not exchanged contacts with the said doctor. It was one of those decisions that you make subconsciously and which somehow turn out to be priceless.

There was a lot of activity at the gate when we arrived at the hospital. You could tell that something was different about that day. More people were walking in and out and even the number of blue dresses that constituted the nurses' uniforms had doubled.

"What's going on here?" we asked the security guard at the gate.

He pointed to a poster that hung on the noticeboard at the gate. We could not believe it! There was a free fistula camp that had been going on for the last three days. That day was the last day of the camp. Doctors had come from all over the country to help carry out corrective surgery for women in the community. The camp was a mobile one, moving from one locality to another.

Ogembo turned to me and we hugged. It was the first time I saw tears roll down his eyes. Walking towards where the visiting doctors had pitched tent, I drove my imagination out of the present moment, and far ahead I could see excitement; a rebirth, the unveiling of a new person, a reason to live and see another day.

A Full Woman

For many communities in 1976 post-colonial Kenya, a woman had no capacity to define herself. As a woman, what defined you was the opinion your husband projected to the society. Womanhood, at the time, had nothing to do with age. At fifteen years of age, I was a woman, although as it were, not a full woman. The other half was lost when I lost my first child. A full woman must have gone full circle, at least once and hold the title 'mother'. I must also have lost some womanhood when apart from losing a child, I lost my life to fistula. Fistula stopped me from living and set me on a path where I walked like a dead person that had just resurrected. From movies, resurrected people wobbled, which was no different from how wobbly my entire life became.

At fifteen, my first husband packed my clothes and asked me to leave his house. At that age, I had no other place to go except back home to my parents. It hurt me very much because it was his child that gave me the fistula. All I knew was that I went to the hospital in labour pains and was operated on, only to wake up with urine and stool leakages with no explanation or management options offered. I was an outcast, rejected by a husband I had been taught to love and neglected by the nurses my life had been entrusted to.

"I cannot stand a girl who urinates on her underpants and stinks my house," were my husband's valedictory words. I had no option but to leave.

It was one thing to be divorced when you were older but it was another when you are just fifteen years old. Apart from becoming the example in the village that other parents used to warn their children not to emulate, you also began to process rejection at a much younger age.

Back at home, very little was discussed about me or my future. Dowry was not paid twice to the same family; therefore, another marriage was not the concern of my parents. As a matter of fact, if I were to be remarried, dowry would be paid to my first husband until such a time that he divorced again, because then it would be concluded that he was the problem.

When a school for the differently-disabled was set up in our village, my father attempted to enrol me.

"Fistula is not a disability," the headteacher of the school told my father.

"It's a disability I tell you," my father struggled to convince him.

"In other words, sir, she is not incapacitated, is she?" he posed.

"This is a log we are staying with. Her smell alone cannot be spread around in the name of walking. She is incapacitated."

The headteacher, sensing my discomfort, sent me out of the office so that they could talk more intensely. It was a god-sent move, not because it saved me the humiliation but because it helped me meet Daniel. Daniel had applied to be a teacher at the school and was scheduled to meet the headteacher that day. He was seated at the waiting room. He liked my smile, he said. We struck up a friendship. We must have talked for about half an hour before I realized that the fellow did not have legs. As a not-so-complete-woman myself, it was funny to see a half-man. I literally laughed and could not have resisted the laughter even if I wanted to. When he realized that I was laughing at him, he joined me in the laughter.

"You are the first person who has not made fun of me behind my back," he said.

That was the beginning of our love story. I was eighteen.

Daniel loved me for who I was. He married me with the fistula and never raised an issue about my past. He never talked of my stench or said any negative word about my situation. While others saw it as a case of two social rejects finding comfort in each other, we knew the truth. The first few minutes of our meeting, the minutes we first liked each other, I had no idea that he had no legs, and he did not know how much of a skunk I was.

All was smooth until hell broke loose after we felt ready to add a new member to our family. The first three pregnancies ended up in stillbirths. Those were dark days for us.

"What did you expect? It's not possible for two lame people to give birth to a complete human being," my father once told my husband.

When I fell pregnant for the fourth time, it was decided between Daniel and me that I leave the village after delivery. I stayed in their home, where he would visit me every weekend.

I gave birth to Gloria, who restored our respect in the community.

However, three pregnancies after Gloria also ended in stillbirth. We resolved to end our quest for a bigger family, only for Gloria to pass away at the age of sixteen. The day Gloria died, everything I ever believed in evaporated. It was devastating for both Daniel and me. There was no chance for restoration after that, especially as I could not conceive again due to secondary infertility.

"Daniel, I know you want a child," I approached him one day after serious thought. He did not respond but I knew he wanted a lineage after him. He sang about it, he dreamt about it.

"You have my permission to marry another wife," I told him. I meant it.

He did marry another wife with whom he has two children. His children call me 'mother' and show me as much love as they show their own mother, and to that extent, we are one family.

My husband had to marry someone else, against his wish because we needed children for inheritance, that was something I had long accepted. He did not like it, but choices were very limited. I insisted that he marry someone else; and it saddened me to release him to another woman but it comforted me to know that he was a deserving man.

It was my co-wife who first opened my mind about surgery. She was the one who heard about a VVF (Vesico-Vaginal Fistula) camp on the radio and told me about it.

"I cannot afford to go all the way to Nairobi for the camp. Where shall I even stay?" I asked her when she fronted the idea.

"I have a sister who lives there, she can host you," she said. The camp was free and she persuaded me that it was my best chance to bid farewell to the problem.

I did travel to Nairobi. I did put up at her sister's.

Going to the clinic helped me to realize that fistula was not a one-woman problem. Many women suffered from the same problem. In the ward, I met a huge number of patients who only served to reflect on the burden that Vesico-Vaginal Fistula (VVF) was for many communities. I met women from all over the country. What I also realized was that many of the women who suffered from the problem gave birth at home, with the common problem being that when things went south, the relatives or persons handling them did not know the correct path to follow.

I was lucky not to mingle a lot with people in my community and escaped much of the public ridicule that I heard the other women went through. In my case, if they called me names, that was up to them but not much broke the wall I had created around me. My life revolved around my family and I had kept it at that.

For me, while leaking urine was a big challenge, losing seven pregnancies was what I never recovered from. Any way I looked at it, there was no way I could keep Daniel to myself after Gloria departed, even when my heart still longed for him. As difficult as it sounded, the decision had to be made. It was my way of saying thank you for his love, warmth, understanding, care and patience through the years.

That was what was running in my mind after my surgery was marked successful in my last check-up. My entire life from 1976 unfolded in my mind. Thirty-eight years of a problem I did not ask for, did not know how to get rid of and that had brought me great love from a man I possibly would never have met. All of that was swept away in one surgery, by one doctor, much younger than myself, born after I had seen a little of the world.

What did not escape my mind too in that journey was the number of herbs I had to chew in their rawness, to boil and drink, to burn and lick their ash, to no avail.

The fact that I did not pay a cent to send the problem away left me with the question why, thirty-eight years ago, the same could not have been done.

As I walked off the bus, heading home to my husband, I felt like other women. Despite not having a child, despite the trouble that I had had to experience, I walked home as a full woman, with the understanding that in all these years, I had always been a full woman, deprived of that title by a society that had deprived me of my whole life.

Battling Stigma

Background

Stigma is the single-most impactful result of low awareness levels among people in the community. While the causatives for stigma share a direct link to community perceptions and influence, this book has opted to separate the two in view of the magnitude of stigma as an independent problem. A lot of women that are affected by fistula and stillbirth are not necessarily isolated by the community, instead they isolate themselves from the community. Even after surgery, some women have no place to call home – raising the need for social reintegration or income-generating activities. This is the first step towards empowerment.

The burden that the women carry makes them brand themselves as social misfits, just as much as they are branded the same. Even those that have been able to manage the condition and desire to reintegrate in the society have challenges fitting in, especially because there is a gap in support programmes for such women after surgery.

The absence of counselling initiatives and awareness campaigns that support the understanding of the issues further push these women into the underbelly of stigma. The narratives in this section offer insights into exactly what this means for the women.

A Dead Life

As I hanged the rope on the tree, created the noose and tested it to see if a human neck could fit into that concentrated space, I began to laugh uncontrollably. In another life, I thought to myself, I would have been an undertaker, or a professional hangman, the kind that governments hire to execute incorrigible death row fellows. The idea that one can make at least one consequential decision in their life, especially when every decision ever made in the process of being alive had had no significant optimistic consequence, was exciting to me.

I laughed even louder when I noticed that the rope was too close to the ground and any attempt to die was likely to fail dramatically.

"The truth is I cannot fail in life then fail to die," I told the rope; then laughed again!

The quiet that followed my insistent laughter was summarily dismissed by a familiar cold movement down the hem of my new skirt, journeying through an improvised corridor on my thighs, through my knees, through my peculiarly hairy legs, and finally into my new pair of socks that soaked the urine well before making contact with my new pair of shoes.

"Not again!" I yelled, but not too loud. Deep down, I knew too well that I was not scared of death. I was prepared for it. The thought that urine had conspired to posthumously suggest to the world that I was the coward who could not face death without peeing on myself, was simply too disturbing. Of course, there had to be a culprit and I did not have to look too far. The blocked catheter with urine seeping from its sides momentarily sprung me back to reality. I was too preoccupied with dying to notice how full my bladder felt, or the empty catheter bag. While I was prepared to die, I was not prepared to die smelling of urine and risk rejection in heaven as the world had shown me on earth.

Quickly, I concealed the rope around one of the branches of the tree and rushed back to my small *makuti* house, a basic structure made of sun-dried coconut palm leaves, common to those of us who had no idea what money smelt like.

Tumaini was still snoring when I opened the door. I did not look at her; I did not have the courage to. Stealthily tiptoeing past her, I reached for the curtain that separated the otherwise one-room structure and headed for my clothes rack. I pulled out another set of new clothes, and a new pair of socks, a just-in-case alternative, for I had planned to die in new clothes – to die clean and wanted, for I had lived dirty and unwelcome.

Back outside, the catheter fixed, I looked for a strong branch to hold on to while climbing the tree, which fell apart with just a little weight applied. I reached for another branch, and up the tree, I tightened the noose around my neck. It was time to jump!

"Watch over Tumaini, Father," I said my last words just as I had planned.

Out of the clear calm that very moment, what I feared most presented itself right before me. Tumaini's voice broke the calm and I gazed down. There she was, crawling towards me, crying.

"Mama … mama … milk…," she said, or rather, struggled to say repetitively.

Embarrassed that my daughter had been punished by the humiliating sight of her mother on the verge of 'euthanasia', I came down the tree, slowly! My only comfort was that she was only two years old and anyway, what did a two-year-old know about a rope on someone's neck?

My maternal instinct prevailed and I gently held her in my arms, slipped my breast out and began to breastfeed her. The crying stopped. I caressed her hair tenderly, knowing well enough that any moment now, she would fall asleep and I would proceed to accomplish my mission. I had to die!

However, as fate would have it, my mother, who had gone to the shopping centre, walked in only to see the rope around my neck with the baby suckling innocently, unaware of what was happening to her mother.

Caught in the shame, I could tell just how heartbroken my mother was when she realized what was happening. She broke into tears but did not say a word. Instead, she hugged me tightly. While I always was aware of her love, that hug was the closest I had ever come to truly feeling something that deeply, at least in the last ten years since fistula became part of my life.

Not a word about what happened was mentioned, not between my mother and me and never to an outsider.

That cold afternoon we however agreed with my mother that by the time my husband got back home by nightfall, I would be far away, far from home.

I arrived at Pastor Anthony's church in the small Islam-dominated island of Lamu a few minutes after sunset. Pastor was a childhood friend of my mother. Although they shared extreme differences with regard to religion, my mother a Muslim and Pastor a Christian who even had a flock of his own to lead, they had remained great friends. As a result, it was easy to feel genuine welcome when Pastor Anthony and his wife opened the front door to their massive church-funded home and led me straight to the dining table for what would be the first serious meal I had had in three days.

Pastor's Anthony's wife took Tumaini and led her to one of the rooms to sleep. I was shown to the bathroom to change clothes and dismiss the urine smell that I carried around me almost all the time.

When I left the bathroom and joined them in the dining area, Pastor Anthony said, "This will be your home for some time." He had a smile on his face.

"Thank you," I responded.

"How long have you had...," he muttered, referring to my situation which I understood my mother had used as bait for them to sympathize just enough to host me.

"For long," I said without intending to commit to any clear answer that would obviously generate undesired sympathy.

"And you are under assistance?"

"I can take care of myself," I affirmed.

"Of course!"

That evening at Pastor's place, a new front in my life opened.

Ten years back the same day, a date that refused to leave my mind, I was in my last week of pregnancy, looking forward to the birth of my child. Some months back, I had just gotten married, traditionally, to my husband Omari. I did not know much about Omari. I had only seen him a few times in the village and what was even funnier was that I first spoke to him on the day of our union. Mine was the case of paying a debt my father owed their family, one that was now due. He had asked to hire their land for five years during the planting seasons to support the university fee payment of my elder brother. He had then just concluded his teaching course and had not immediately found a job to begin the process of debt repayment. Therefore, something had to be done about the debt. I happened to be what had to be given to one of their sons who was now ripe for marriage. They could also see that I was ripe. I was only sixteen!

I became expectant almost immediately after the marriage. The birth of a child was apparently urgent to the family as Omari's mother had begun to suffer an illness that many community healers had concluded would not give her much time to be alive. As they also advised, she could afford nine months, and another nine months perhaps where she would be able to see and bless at least two grandchildren. My brief was to churn out as many children as I could within the shortest time possible.

To support the realization of this goal, Omari's mother, who was now my mother-in-law, ruled our marriage with an iron fist. To put it bluntly, she would ask me every morning if I had had sex with my husband. She even went as far as suggesting some of the possible sex routines that could lead to pregnancy at an efficient speed and which she duly demonstrated in the most visual of ways.

Her advice worked. I became pregnant, a pregnancy that she also micromanaged – from what I ate, to how many hours I could sleep, to the kind of activities I could engage in (hard labour was her preference): because I could not give birth to a weak child.

One month to my due date, she summoned me and commanded that I should not have sex any more until the king arrived from my womb. It was determined through her own observation that the child I was expecting was a boy. She had already settled on her late husband's name for the child.

The problem with her command was that it was directed to the wrong person. I did not even like sex myself. It was an exercise I could do anything to run away from given a chance. On the other hand,

Omari was excited about sex. He had formed a habit of taking brief breaks at work at any time during the day and rushing home. Mostly, I would be seated outside the house with the other women discussing our husbands in graphic details. He would then call me into the house and demand that I have sex with him. To him, I was a sex object. He did not value preparation; I was supposed to always be ready. He did not even talk to me or consider that at the very least, I was pregnant.

"Lie down...! Turn...! Bend...!" he would order ... no feelings attached, no respect or regard to my situation. It did not matter to him whether I liked it or not, whether I was in pain or not ... he would lay with me and then just go. I guess it must have been decided that my father's debt had to be paid the hard way.

In this regard, my mother-in-law's command landed on the wrong ears, because sex had to go on for Omari, when and how he liked it.

One week to my due date on a Sunday morning, Omari's mother arrived at our door at 6 o'clock in the morning while he was sweating on top of me. She pushed the door open since the *makuti* houses did not have permanent doors.

Seeing as we were in that state, she came in, held Omari's bare buttocks firmly in her hands and pulled him away from me. She then firmly held his manhood in her left hand as she slapped the life out of me. "You are busy being mounted at this time like chicken? Stop it right now and get out of this home you sick woman. During my time I never used to be mounted all the time," she howled, blaming me for the situation.

That day, I decided that I had had enough. I left for my parents' house that morning – empty handed. Neither Omari nor his mother followed up to know what happened to me. My parents, on the other hand, were disappointed that I could not keep something as simple as a marriage together.

"How weak a woman are you?" my father would often ask.

"As a woman, when you are beaten, you say thank you and move on with life," my mother advised.

I lived with my parents until labour started. The labour itself was a nightmare and it ended up crushing me for two days, forcing my parents, whose original plan was to have me deliver at home with the help of a midwife, to take me to the hospital for delivery. We then left for the District Hospital together with my mother where I was examined several times. They finally decided to take me for a Caesarean section operation. At the time, the baby was well, he was playing … I could feel his movements just as usual. The only issue that was raised by the healthcare providers was that the baby's passage was small, but the baby was okay.

In the theatre, I was given anesthesia before the surgery. I did not make good progress. For some reason, I kept falling in and out of sleep for what I was later told was five days. When I recovered, I found myself in the ward, alone. I had expected to see my baby right beside me, but he was not there.

My mother walked in just as I was still familiarizing myself with my surrounding. Behind her was a nurse, the one that received me when I was brought in.

"She died!" my mother broke the news.

"She…? Who is 'she'?" I asked, confused.

"The child died. She died!"

"Whose child?" I retorted.

My mother at this point seemed to think that I was not fully aware of myself yet. I was! Except that my child was a boy. This was a mistake, I thought. I protested on those grounds.

"It was a girl and she's dead," the nurse declared with finality.

It was at that time that I also felt something between my legs. I slowly moved my hands to examine what had happened to me.

"Careful!" advised the nurse.

"What is this?" I asked.

"A catheter," she said and added that it should remain *in situ*, otherwise there would be consequences. As though the death of my child was not painful enough, I now had the realization that something new had taken over my body, a fistula … whatever that was!

According to our culture, the baby was to be buried at my husband's home. Omari did not have a problem with that. However, my mother-in-law was convinced that I had hidden her son's baby boy and bought a dead baby girl from unscrupulous dealers at the hospital, which I was now handing over to them for burial. She stood her ground – against custom.

We buried the child beside my paternal grandfather's grave. Neither Omari nor his mother showed up for the burial.

Pastor Anthony who had probed me to tell them the story stopped me at this point.

"Is he the one you have run away from? Omari?" he asked.

"Yes," I said.

After I left the hospital, I lived with my parents for two years. Then out of the blue, my mother-in-law came begging me to return to my matrimonial home. I have never understood what motivated her to do that. When she died a week after her visit, it was again decided for me that we could not disrespect the dying wish of an old person. That began the unregulated cycle of violence that I now had to live with. It was also during that time that Tumaini was born.

"What has made you run away?" Pastor Anthony's wife asked.

"I am tired," I said with tears rolling out of my eyes.

At that moment, I heard Tumaini cry. Pastor Anthony's wife went to hold her. She brought her to where we were.

"She is a beautiful baby," she said.

We turned our eyes to Tumaini. She had suddenly turned from crying to laughing. We also laughed at how fast the switch happened, only to realize that she was pointing at my legs. I was dripping urine. Embarrassed, I stood up.

"Sit," said Pastor Anthony.

I sat down, uncomfortably. It was the first time someone had actually not expressed disgust for messing their property. I had lived a life full of feelings of dejection, cohabiting with a man who had no positive emotions or respect for me. All I dealt with were rejection, poverty, stigmatization, stress, continuous urine leakage, lack of diapers, suicidal tendencies, gender violence and homelessness. So, to be told to sit down with my urine on a seat was both uncomfortable and touching.

"What if we told you that we could help you?" asked Pastor Anthony, almost bordering on the rhetorical.

"I have tried everything, every herb there is to try, Pastor," I said.

"Not herbs. A doctor…! Surgery," he added.

"I can't afford that," I said.

"That will be up to us."

"Are you sure?" I asked, breaking down.

"Yes, I was treated for the same. I got healed," Pastor Anthony's wife chipped in.

"Healed? One can heal?" I was taken aback.

Pastor Anthony's wife led me to the guest bedroom. I would wake up a new woman, she said, then switched off the lights and left the room. I stared into the ceiling blankly. I did not know what to do or to think, but I knew at that moment what was furthest from my mind was what has been closest for ten years ... suicide!

One Way or the Other

I smiled for the first time. It was at the thought of death. How did I not think of it earlier? Why would anyone suffer in this world when they could sleep sweetly forever? I pinched myself for having not thought of it before. Death is the most effective option of overcoming problems of the world. How sweet, how easy! I smiled again, I was going to the other world, to start a fresh life. A new life with better decisions. A better life far from my family. But even death is very proud. It hates the poor just like life hates the poor. A pauper is always at the border of life and death, but neither wants the pauper. As such, suffering gladly chooses the poor, to maul and harass at will. Dying, as I realized, needed money too. A poor person cannot afford a quick death. I had no cent to buy a hanging rope. Neither did I have some to purchase poison.

My friend Kerubo would joke often that 'beer is thicker than blood' and we would laugh it away. I never imagined I would experience it first-hand.

"Is this our Deborah?" my sister asked in a tone of mixed disbelief and disgust.

Her eyes keenly inspected me, travelling from my colourless face to my big stomach to the hospital bedding.

"Debo!" my mother called, her red eyes piercing me with contempt.

"I sent you to school to open your brain and earn a certificate, but you decided to open your legs for men and earn yourself fistula. Your problem!" she added with finality.

They did not care that I had lost a child. In fact, their reason for visiting was to make an official statement that shame was a personal responsibility. It was not a family matter that they were willing to be part of. I was to carry my shame alone.

Mother was an untraditional woman, a hopeless drunkard. She often proclaimed to be the chief alcohol tester in any new drinking den in the village. She would then spread the word around amongst fellow drunkards, a review of the quality of alcohol. While she admonished me at the hospital bed, the smell of cheap liquor escaping her mouth hit my nose violently. She belched severally and forcefully, always at the verge of throwing up where I lay. I was sure she would not have been remorseful had she done so. Through her tired and condescending face, an indifferent though angered tone, I could feel that she may even have considered it a huge favour to break from her drinking duties to see a worthless daughter in hospital.

"You are a walking curse, young fool," she relieved the words from her mind and left.

I prepared my apologies as I anticipated their next visit, hoping they would be less angry and more forgiving. It was a terribly bad feeling to be the black sheep in the family. Ironically, my own mother had imported enough shame into the house to last us three lifetimes. If she was ever to choose between us, me especially, and her alcohol, she would embrace her bottle unapologetically.

Days gave in to weeks, my eyes stubbornly remained fixed at the door, hoping to see my sisters or drunk mother crawl in. I was ready to endure their abuse and rebuke, but I broke at the reality of their absence. Nobody would leave a fourteen-year-old girl in a hospital bed alone. Only the foolish Bosco would do that. Bosco was two classes ahead of me. A short and dark coward, with a nose thrice bigger than the ordinary size. How did a person that foolish live so comfortably among people? How did such a big-nosed hyena succeed in inflating my stomach for nine months in the name of love? I mused with bitterness. I cringed at the memory of his denial of the pregnancy.

"I have never seen this girl in my entire life!" Bosco swore before his mother.

The loss of my child and the memory of his betrayal shattered me. It paralysed me more as the weeks grew into months and my mother and sister had not yet reappeared.

"Did they come while I was asleep?" I asked the nurse.

"They? Who?"

"My mother and sister."

"No, get some rest, they will come," she would reply pitifully.

Maybe they had no money, maybe they were still angry, I pondered.

In the ward, Mama Prisca did not like me. She did not want me to look at her child.

"You will transfer your bad spirits to my child," she would say.

Her sharp malicious tongue influenced many to share her venomous beliefs. Several imagined that a woman who had had a stillbirth would transfer the bad luck to their children, and they too would die. It was crushing to hear them whisper to one another that they should cover their babies so that my eyes would not fall on them. The babies' cries reminded me of my own who never cried nor saw the world like the rest did. I often imagined how beautiful her cry would be. Her soft touches as she held tenderly to me, struggling to empty my breasts. I would smile at her as she slept. The images of how she would have been, were she to breathe, would keep me awake all night, smiling, crying. The bittersweet imagination would only be broken by the painful thoughts of my family's betrayal. Their absence was too loud.

"Your leg is much better now; I can organize to take you home," Nurse Mwende pronounced, ending my six-month confinement at the hospital that was the result of nerve damage on my left leg. I had accumulated a huge bill at the time. Luckily for me, an investigative piece recently carried out by one of the major media houses in the country, exposing the plight of people detained in hospital due to their inability to cater for bills, had sparked a huge public outcry that made it possible for us to be let go without any demands – at least until the public forgot again.

"Home? NO!" I protested.

I would rather have remained in the hospital than gone back to my mother's house. A mother that would choose beer over her child was not a mother.

I resolved to go to my married sister's place.

As soon as I arrived, the entrance of the house was marked by urine leaking on my sister's hand-woven carpet. I had felt something strangely familiar roll down my thighs. The problem with it was that it never announced that it wanted out. Neither did it resist the commands of my bladder. It just came out when and how it wanted to; a disturbing reminder of the other misfortune that I had earned at the hospital – the curse that was fistula.

The shock on my sister's face was one I had never seen on any other human being.

"Debo! Are you mad? Why did you not ask where the toilet is! Does my house look like some bush where you just stand and urinate in like a drunkard?"

"I am sorry!" I apologized, shaking with shame.

Her children stood at a safe distance, inspecting, wondering, disbelieving. How could a big girl urinate on herself senselessly! Their father, like most men, silently peered at me from the corners of an old newspaper he was reading when I came into the house. He chose to nurse his shock quietly rather than join in the melodrama of his short wife.

"Debo! Decide if you came to urinate or to live in this house, you will rot my mattresses!" Nyageso, my sister, shouted one day after I wet my bed for the third day in a row.

I was helpless. The many layers of clothing I had added in my panties to prevent leakage did not stop the rebellious urine. Furthermore, the odour that was also my trademark attracted so much bile from my sister. Her children had privately vowed never to sit close to me. Whenever I passed close to them, they would jump away as if they were about to step on faeces accidentally. Or they would simply hold their noses. The humiliation was prodigious but I could not blame them. They were innocent in their reaction. Children always express themselves truthfully and they would never consciously show contempt.

When our sister Kerubo paid us a visit, she loudly announced that I should not go near her or wear her clothes.

"I do not want to smell like raw sewage and gift my smooth skin with foreign diseases and rashes!" she said.

I got used to the humiliation. I was used to the contemptible invectives. I could ignore the abuse of strangers, distant relatives who called me *amache esosera* (stagnant rainwater), but I could not endure the vileness and contempt from my very blood. It was terrible. I felt worthless. Family was my world, my last resort, but that world had abused me when I was defenseless. It was at that time that I smiled at the thought of suicide. I did not understand why they gave it such a crude name. Suicide sounded salty, yet in reality, it was sweet. It was an end to pain, an end to shame and an end to loneliness.

When Mariamu, my sister's house-help heard about my wishes, she was not shocked. She was disappointed that I had affirmed what she always heard.

"You are a fool. A foolish fool. I am disappointed. I had always doubted when they called you scatterbrain...," Mariamu said as she looked at me condescendingly.

"Instead of looking for a job as a house-help and saving the money to seek treatment, here you are fantasizing about death," she added.

But it was better to just die. Mariamu did not understand. She was not with me as I suffered the humiliation and heartbreak, hopping from one home to another, being dismissed after a month, a week and sometimes not even going beyond the interview. Other times, I left without pay, enduring painful months on end as punishment for wetting their beds and couches. She was not with me when Mama Clarissa sent me to the shop only to come back to find a padlock at the gate and the two pieces of cloth that were my wealth thrown outside. No, she did not understand me. All she did was abuse a suffering girl who only wanted a fresh life in the other world. How heartless! Why would anyone wish another person pain and humiliation when they would have been happier when dead?

It rained heavily that night. It was also my second week working as a house-help for Miss Wamumbi in Kitale town where I had gone hunting for another job, a strange land where nobody knew me. While laying the table for dinner, it happened again. She clicked violently, throwing her hands in the air.

"I am tired! Go rain outside."

She threw me out of her house, terming my leakage as rainwater. I was also tired. It was pointless trying to live in a world that constantly battered you. If a vehicle ran over me properly, I would die of shock before the pain kicked in. All I needed to do was to properly position myself by the roadside then jump on the road when the vehicle was at close range. I would not choose just any car. A slow car may have ended up just injuring and breaking a few bones, earning me another long life of suffering with an additional title – a cripple. It had to be a speeding car that would crush me instantly, severing my bones and my soul in one shot.

Standing by the roadside for several minutes, waiting for the perfect car to drive by, I did not realize that someone behind me was staring at me. Our eyes interlocked just as I was giving the world a final look with the perfect one in sight, a few metres away.

"Are you going somewhere?" he asked.

"Yes. Home!"

"Hold my hand. I will take you home."

Today, many months later as we walked to the hospital to replace my catheter, passing the same spot we met, I looked at my husband Luke who was by my side and smiled.

"What's amusing you my dear?" he asked.

"Nothing," I smiled.

A New Life, a Rising Sun

She is sixty-six, but can pass for forty. Her ebony skin, though slightly wrinkled, covers a slender frame that could have been broader with a better diet. Her high cheekbones could easily have turned her into a strong candidate for the likes of Peter Beard – the man who discovered legendary models including Naomi Campbell.

At her age, Peninnah Mwende has learnt to live with disappointments and celebrate the little gifts that life presents. She interacts with people of all age groups, with her sense of humour leaving roars of laughter in her wake.

"I care less," she quips at young men who have now stopped to draw from her endless pot of witty jokes. "You are the sons that I never had, after all. All of you are my sons. When you go home, please pass my regards to your folks. Tell them that your grandmother who once peed like chicken, sent you." She does not disappoint.

They all seem to know her story. Mwende is a common figure at the Mbaikini Market, in Machakos' Wamunyu area. Wamunyu is known in Kenya for its famous wood carvings that continue driving the curio sector in Kenya. The area is also one of the driest parts of Lower Eastern Kenya, where the Kamba community have recorded some of the most celebrated milestones in the Kenyan political and academic spheres.

Beside the big names and acts of Wamunyu, Mwende sits deftly at the apex of the social fabric of Wamunyu, having been among the few women who inherited land from their fathers. For a community whose life is steeped in patriarchal cultural and social norms, hers is a very unique case, which draws mixed opinion. However, the general consensus favours Mwende. Most locals aver that any father would have done what her dad did for his daughter. Mwende has endured the worst that life has thrown on her laps.

"You are laughing at this *susu* (grandmother) because of her age? See, I can pull all the moves that would shame your ever half-naked girlfriends," she says and breaks into a silly dance.

"One, two, three, four!

Get up, (get on up)

Get up, (get on up)
Stay on the scene, (get on up), like a sex machine, (get on up),"

She sings the famous song by the godfather of Soul, James Brown. There is more laughter, as young men join in. They all love Mwende.

Despite her age and lanky frame, Mwende is a tomboy. She can ride bicycles, drive cars with a shift gear and herd livestock like a man. At the age of fifteen, she had learnt how to drive sand trucks behind her father's back. He learnt about it the day she drove off for over twenty kilometres with some police officers who had tried to arrest her. They jumped and ran off when she threatened to drive the darn lorry into a river. Her father was forced to part with a five hundred shilling bribe to settle the issue. It is also claimed that in her childhood, Mwende loved watching goats mate.

She recently returned to Mbaikini from her latest medical sojourn in Nairobi, where she had been for almost three weeks. Many locals are used to her trips. They know her. They have seen her run around the village, stinking and dripping with urine. Many have discussed her in both hushed and loud tones. She knows them too. She softly claps back through her often-ribald jokes. So used are locals to Mwende's medical issue, that they now see her as a copybook of witty flaw … No one is perfect, they say. She no longer smells or drips urine but her current status never came easy.

Twenty-five years ago, Mwende was a happily married woman. Her husband, Boniface Mutisya, was a man at peace, having secured himself the love of his life – a beautiful girl who could mount a tiger. She could guide the donkey to the well, teach his brother's children to ride bicycles and work on the family farm like the beasts of burden she rode. That was until she landed in her messy twenty-five-year trap.

Memories still fresh … mangoes were in season, and this being Mwende, climbing a tree while five months pregnant was nothing odd. While busy breaking taboos once again, she missed a step, slipped and then went tumbling down like a ripe mango that could no longer hold on.

"I felt a sharp pain that cut from below my belly all the way to my back. I then started bleeding, then screamed like a bush baby," she says.

Her in-laws arrived. They were later joined by her husband, who took her to the nearby Mbaikini Dispensary, five kilometres away. The clinical officer referred her to the then Machakos District Hospital.

"Doctors told me that the foetus had jumped. My belly was massaged until I regretted not miscarrying," she says as a dark cloud of sorrow engulfs her. She was meant to undergo an operation, but her husband had returned home so there was no one to append a signature for consent. By morning, she had lost the baby and was unable to walk.

"They used metal clippers to remove the dead foetus. This might have punctured me internally," Mwende quips. "I walked around like a newly-circumcised boy, with legs wide apart," she adds and breaks into laughter.

Her in-laws visited her in hospital the following day, upon receiving news of her loss. Her mother and father would arrive two days later. It was here that she was taken in for surgery to correct her situation. Six hours later, she was moved to a ward where she came to.

"I realized that I was wallowing in pee. I was wet from my waist downwards. I believe my buttocks were seared by my sourish pee. I thought my sexual organs were rotten," she adds as she laughs heartily. It then dawned on her that she could not control her urine. When her mother-in-law returned to the hospital, she was the first to notice it.

She turned to her son and said, "You need to move on now. This woman cannot be of help to you in any way. I don't think the damage is repairable." She bitterly adds, "His mother was telling her son to abandon me in my time of need. Some mothers-in-law are manufactured in hell!"

From then on, no one from her husband's side of the family paid her a visit. They left her to her own devices, amid hostile hospital staff who demanded that she pay and vacate her bed for other patients.

Her father was concerned. He went to her father-in-law's home and complained vociferously. He was fed up. He demanded his daughter's belongings so that he could take care of her. To him, they were mere honkers. That was how she ended up at home, living with her parents. That was also how she bid married life goodbye. Back in her native Mbaikini, word went round that Mwende had abandoned marriage and was now bed-wetting.

"The ridicule was too much. Some said that I had had rough sex with my hubby, leading to my being raptured. Others claimed that I had been bewitched. They even went ahead and suggested that I had disrespected my father-in-law, who cursed me and later chased me out. Some of my childhood friends even suggested that I visit a famous witchdoctor in the neighbouring Kitui County, and even Tanzania."

She underwent three surgeries at the Machakos Level 5 Hospital. For a while, she could not pass urine. "Doctors were forced to insert tubes into me to allow the liquid to flow," she says.

Even then, she did not have control of her bowels. Her father was running low on finances. He sold the remaining goats and cows to finance yet another surgery at the then Embu Provincial Hospital. It was there that she was informed that she had a fistula. Doctors there also revealed to her that she may not bear any more children.

"I had never heard of fistula in my entire life, until it started wreaking havoc between my thighs. My first attempt at motherhood ended up being my last," she dejectedly concludes.

After the last surgery, Mwende landed at the local market, where she sold foodstuffs. This proved to be a challenge since she still could not control her urine. She was sanguine about it and openly spoke about her condition to her fellow traders. Some condemned her, while others empathized. She still maintained her sense of humour and would use her case to poke fun at herself to the amusement of her colleagues. Some even thought of her as one of the mad people who are a common feature in some African flea markets.

Locals later embraced her and often came to her defence whenever anyone mocked her. Some even dedicated themselves to buying from her, just to support her.

One day, a client noticed her condition and advised that she visit Kenyatta National Hospital, but Mwende was too broke to travel to Nairobi. Her colleagues organised a mini funds drive that saw her attend a clinic at the referral hospital. There, she underwent yet another operation that dragged on for eight hours.

"I went to hell and back. I saw all manner of visions, good and bad. What remains etched in me, was a vision of a man tearing a piece of flesh and throwing away the rotten parts. He would then use fresh tissue from a bucket tucked between his legs, and replace the rotten ones with new ones. From the work of his hands, a new face emerged. It then smiled at me and vanished," she says.

"I woke up in a ward. I was freezing. My teeth were chattering as I tried calling out for help. It was like I had just landed from another planet. A nurse came and calmed me down. She then walked away and returned after a few minutes, accompanied by a man. That was the doctor. He smiled and told me that I was one lucky soul. He added that I had to be resuscitated three times during the marathon operation. It is also here that he told me that they had redirected my urine to my rectum. Hence my peeing like a chicken," she adds as she laughs.

She was, however, advised against holding urine whenever she felt the urge to visit the toilet. That was how she survived for three years.

One evening, on her way home from Mbaikini market, she witnessed an interesting accident. A rickshaw had just lost control and crashed in a ditch. Locals were rescuing the occupants. The first to be pulled out of the wreckage was the rider. Then the passenger emerged. He had wet his pants! Mwende laughed her head off.

"I know it was silly, but I realized why people made fun of me. It is quite hilarious seeing an adult in wet pants. It was even funnier, the shaken man in a well-cut suit, with what appeared like map of urine below his crotch. The wet patch was interesting," she confesses.

The man did not seem to notice it. She approached him and innocently asked him if he also had a fistula like her. That rattled the passenger into reality. He turned to her and asked her how she knew about fistula.

"I just told him that I acquired it when I miscarried," she says.

It turned out that the man was a clinical officer at the Kenyatta National Hospital. He was visiting a friend in Mbaikini and was on his way back to the main terminus to catch a public service vehicle to Nairobi when the accident happened. Anyway, local rickshaw operators are known to be a crafty lot with a special liking for cheap liquor. The thuggish characters are also responsible for the number of children born to teenage girls in the area. Any parent with a school-going daughter is not fond of the perps.

As she bantered with the confused passenger, the chap handed her a business card and walked away, after requesting her to call him after two days.

After cheekily apologizing for wetting his pants in public, the clinical officer asked her to travel to Nairobi the following week. There was a medical camp for women with fistula and she could benefit from it. Again, the traders came through for her. Three days later, she was in the elevator with the man, whose name she could not pronounce, as they headed to the clinic. She was screened and later given a number.

Her stint in the theatre lasted for four hours. She came to in a noisy ward.

"It was like a mental asylum. I found myself amongst several women, some wailing while others were grunting in pain. There was this girl who was clearly afflicted. She kept shouting a man's name, cursing him for putting her in her mess. I clearly understood her."

Euphrates Masakhalia passed by. That was the man who had informed Mwende about the clinic. The man whose name she could not pronounce.

"It has been two planting seasons without me wetting my panties, or passing urine through my anus. This is a miracle. If I had a daughter, I would advise her to pursue a course in medicine, to be like those fine doctors. I would also push her to marry that man with a difficult name," she says laughing.

She also calls upon the society to be mindful of the plight of women with fistula.

"I coped through humour. But deep down, I was crumbling. How many women have resolve like mine?" she asks.

As the sun turns gold as it settles in the west, Mwende stumbles on her way home, walking with a steady brisk pace. Life is always a rising sun.

My Flaws, Flows and the Hope that Lies in Science

"You better act like an adult or I finish you off like your coward Bairege warriors. The miscreants cannot even separate two fighting chicks," my husband snarled as he landed yet another mighty slap on my cheek. Blood splattered from my lower lip.

"A whole adult woman who pees and excretes on herself is a disgrace," he added. Another uppercut slap from him jerked me to the opposite side.

I could not believe that things had slumped to this. My Julian Chacha hitting me like a slave? How things changed…

"Julian, you know very well that I haven't been this way until we lost the baby …" I beseeched him.

"We lost the baby? Who are 'we'? You lost the baby when you turned into a toddler. That was the last stroke. You lost my only son who could have upheld my legacy. That is the boy who could have held us together. Just as he is gone, so are we!" he growled as his massive kick landed on my right thigh.

Immediately, I felt a stream of my shame run down my inner thigh onto the floor. The stench filled the living room as my four young daughters scampered.

I was not hurt by the beatings. Rather, the fact that my Julian was hitting me for the umpteenth time, and making me feel like the scum that I was. I had allowed it for the last three years. This was my way of keeping him. But it seemed like it was as good as drawing water in a gunny bag. My stench was driving him further and further away from me. He had brought in another woman with two sons from a previous marriage. My previously happy home was turned into a nightmare as I was constantly harassed and harangued by the new family over my flawed flows. He had joined them. One evening, I could not take it any more.

I lost it and engaged the woman in the mother of all fights. We fought well. She must have underestimated my strength, because I gave her a thorough thrashing that left her with a broken leg. I later threw her and her nasty boys out. When Julian returned in the evening, our

Kuria elders stood by me. They ordered him to find another place for his second wife, if he indeed was keen on being polygamous. But he was ordered to continue providing for us, just like any other man keen on expanding his harem. He joined them, only to return and assault me. He was revenging the daily provisions by battering me.

This time, I decided to draw the line. He was either mine or not. So as my murk flowed on the floor, he walked out, spat and then pensively stared at the ground. I wobbled around, holding my kicked, aching thigh to the door. I leaned on the frame and muttered, "Such a warrior who has descended from the heroics of the battlefields to assaulting women he claims to love …"

I must have touched a raw nerve. Julian swerved his huge, stout frame and charged at me. I took off and locked myself in the bedroom. He almost broke the door. I was prepared to meet my maker, until the moment I heard him walk out, his heavy steps pounding the floor. I kept myself locked in the room.

"Useless woman. My warrior son married a woman who pees and defecates in her groin. Has he finished you?" That was my mother-in-law. I was used to her insults. She had always been against me from the day she learnt that I was from the Bairege clan. She never had peace, after learning that her warrior son was eyeing a girl from the enemy clan. She grudgingly accepted this after elders from both Bairege and Banyabasi clans convinced her that our marriage would bring peace between the two ever-warring sides. We had been living under a shaky peace until three years ago, until the hole in me widened the gap. The hole that was the source of my torment. Mother's incessant insults and shaming epithets still haunt me. I have never found peace nor the urge to forgive her. Hopefully, one day, I will.

A huge crack had developed between me and Julian when I fell pregnant for the fifth time, in 1990. There were no scans to tell the gender of the baby, but I hoped against hope that it would be a boy. Before that, I had some few issues with Julian, apparently for piling girls in his space. Julian did not speak directly to me on this, but his mother would castigate me for not giving the Banyabasi clan a son to carry on her son's fighting legacy. I did not expect my Julian to give in to the social pressure, since he was an educated man. I was clearly deceiving myself.

One evening, Julian failed to return home from work. The evening turned into a week. Although we worked in the same ministry, his office was in a different building. I later barged in on him one afternoon with another woman, in a tight embrace. When I demanded answers, he calmly turned to me and said, "Angela Boke, you have a co-wife. I need a son and I found the perfect person to help me achieve that." I was stupefied. He had never called me by my full name until that day.

The following weekend, he brought the woman out. She had two sons from her previous relationships. They were aged eight and six years. From then henceforth, I became a stranger in my house. The woman would set her boys against my daughters, leading to ugly altercations between us, while my Julian did nothing about it.

The evening when we had fought, I had found that my things had been moved into my children's bedroom. She had changed my bedroom curtains and moved her sons into the guest bedroom, while I was supposed to sleep with my four daughters. My first-born daughter was bleeding from the nose after being assaulted by the elder boy. I flipped. I attacked her. We fought for over one hour as my mother-in-law cheered her on. I later turned the tide against her. I beat her to a pulp. I grunted with satisfaction as her femur snapped under my weight. Mother screamed. My victim was dragged to the hospital. I moved my stuff back to my marital bedroom and threw hers together with her boys' out. When Julian returned home late that evening, he tried to order me out of the house. I called one of his uncles, who arrived accompanied by the three Kuria elders. They were the ones who ordered Julian to take care of his new woman, and continue supporting us. However, he would only come once in a while, perform his marital obligations but demean me.

My antenatal records were clean, until the ninth month. One day, while heading home from my last visit to the clinic, I felt dizzy, but the feeling later passed. On arriving home, I took a bed rest. Later in the evening, as I prepared to go to bed, my water broke. Immediately, I felt the dizziness once again, before bleeding kicked in. Within no time, the placenta came out. That was shocking. I had had three normal deliveries before, yet had never witnessed a placenta precede the baby. However, my fourth girl was born through Caesarean section.

My daughters called their father from my co-wife's home, and he later took me to the Kehancha Hospital. He also thought that it was my due date. I kept telling him that the whole issue was odd, but he kept reassuring me that all would be well.

I was admitted in a ward. At around 6 p.m., I was prepared and taken to the theatre. That was when I sensed danger. Doctors performed a C-section on me and removed the baby. When I regained my strength, the doctor on duty came to my bed and told me that I had had a baby boy, who had unfortunately passed away. I was jarred. I kept my emotional torment to myself until the following morning. There were no cell phones back then.

I only informed Julian when he came visiting me the following morning. He was gutted. He cried in the wards and started blaming the doctors for failing to save his only son. He became violent and was sedated before being sent to the male ward.

The following morning, he walked into the ward, now calm and assured me that all was well. He later left and returned with my co-wife, our mother-in-law and other relatives. The infant's body was taken away, after I refused to view it. After all, my son was dead.

A medical report from the hospital indicated that my son's head was blocked by my left leg, making it hard to pass through the pelvic bones to reach the vaginal opening. He suffocated and died due to lack of oxygen. Doctors did not know what had led to this. But the report also indicated that I had had prolonged labour. They tried resuscitating him after delivery in vain.

Upon being discharged three days later, I did not even ask where they buried the body. However, the death hit me hard. I sank into a depressive state for two weeks. I never wanted to see anyone nursing a baby. Crying babies would rattle me, sending my breast milk to flow like a river. Besides this, I was also battling another issue: the blood clots that were flowing from my vagina. I was also unable to hold my urine. I could not wear any underwear. The clots and urine would soak my panties in seconds. Soon, my urine corroded my bedding, leaving me exposed to the bare bed. I filled up the spaces with old clothes before replacing the bedding after receiving my salary.

Julian, upon realising that I was in a mess, moved out of the house, changed my insurance details and replaced me with his second wife. He also avoided passing by my house. He would assault me for wetting my bed and blame me for the death of his son. He was more fixated on his adoptive sons from his second wife. He completely withdrew from our daughters and would sometimes abuse them for being what he termed 'call girls-in-waiting'.

I went back to the hospital and was referred to the Migori District Hospital. One of the doctors there examined me and said that I had raptured my bladder and part of my rectum during the difficult delivery. He also added that I would need surgery to rectify the matter, which could not be done at the facility. He instead referred me to the Nyanza Provincial Hospital, popularly known as Russia. I managed to go to the hospital after two weeks. By then, the world had started crumbling around me.

Going to work became a difficult issue. I was the git of the office. My colleagues avoided me and complained that I was stinking. My bosses moved me to an abandoned office, where I worked alone, using the telephone to take orders and have any other communication. I was also ridiculed by people sent to me for assistance. Being a clerk in a government institution, it was very hard for me to be sacked, but my bosses put in bad reports about me, leading to an avalanche of warning letters from the ministry headquarters. My husband did nothing to protect me. He acted like a stranger. Eventually, I opted to quit on medical grounds.

At home, my mother-in-law had taken to the habit of coming to my house to hurl degrading words at me, right in front of my daughters. She would blame herself for allowing her son to marry a woman who could not bear him a son. A woman who had even turned herself into a toddler, soiling herself to attract sympathy. One of her sons even proposed that I see a traditional healer to fix my issues with my ancestors. When I refused, he went ahead and brought one to my house in my absence. The sick man decreed that I should be violated for two hours to teach me a lesson.

When I heard about this, I reported the matter to the local police station. From there, I was given police protection. I later moved back home to Ntimaru, in Kuria East, with my daughters. However, I was later forced to go back by my family. Julian, as usual, said and did nothing.

In my Kuria community and specifically amongst the Abairege and Abanyabasi clans, boys are born to be warriors. This is premised on the decades-old animosity between the two clans. The Abanyabasi and Abairege have baffled any outsiders and fellow Kuria clans for long. Other Kuria clans like the Abakira and Abagumbe live peacefully with all other clans, including us. All clans spread all the way into the neighbouring Tanzania. However, Abanyabasi and Abairege have been killing each other with abandon. On a normal day, people from the two clans cannot see eye to eye. The frequent clashes are steeped in cattle rustling. Although Bantu speakers, they raid and kill like nomads.

Whenever theft of livestock is reported in one of the clans, it leads to ugly fights that leave many young men dead. So bad is the situation that locals nowadays share rooms with their prized cows. Young men with murderous teeth are hailed as heroes by their respective clansmen. It is a pious quest to cleanse them of their thirst for spilling innocent blood. Young widows whose husbands die in these pyrrhic fights are celebrated, while being preyed on by the surviving warriors. It is a culture that has bred a knack for young men dancing on each other's graves.

One such warrior is my husband, Julian. On the battlefield, he was as fierce as Napoleon Bonaparte. He swung the AK 47 assault rifle like a Russian mercenary and left the poor Bairege warriors dead in their numbers. Whenever he led the raid, more and more cows would be driven towards Kegonge, leaving families in Ntimaru heaving in grief as they buried their young men. Julian would be celebrated with slaughtered cows and chicken, decorated with flowers and given young girls to soothe his tired loins in the night.

Before Julian's arrival, Abairege warriors tormented the Abanyabasi. They had sharpened their fighting skills from engagements with Kipsigis and Maasai warriors, who live across the ridge in Transmara.

Julian used to lead these raids over the weekend. During weekdays, he was this brilliant class seven pupil at Kegonge primary school. Even after joining secondary school, he still used to lead his peers in attacks during the holidays. He apparently stopped when he joined university and graduated with a degree in education.

I got married to my husband in the early 80s, when he was a teacher at Migori Boys Secondary School. He was later promoted to a senior education officer, based at Kehancha. I worked in the Personnel Department as a junior clerk.

Being from the Abairege clan, his family was opposed to our marriage, until Julian stood his ground, prompting elders from the two clans to step in. However, my mother-in-law seemed to have refused to move on, using my bearing of daughters as a reason to instigate her devious ideas. The stillbirth of my son, and my reeking of faeces and urine however, broke the camel's back.

At the Nyanza General Hospital, I was booked for surgery but it was postponed thrice due to a shortage of experts. By then, my body had begun reacting strangely. I would experience spates of pain that left my chest badly congested. I even thought that the urine and blood clots were moving upwards to my mouth. I lost a lot of weight since I could not eat most solid foods. I survived on a little liquid for fear of escalating the urine flow. I stopped attending church services as I was the target of callous remarks. During the few times that I did, I used to sit far away from the rest and follow the proceedings while struggling to hold the soaked clothes between my thighs. I always sought a vantage point that would allow me to dash to the lavatory with my bag full of linen, change the soggy ones and head home as fast as possible, since I could not return to church with stinking clothes in my bag.

I also quit the choir, quit all women groups and a teenagers' club that I patronized. I watched as my friends shrunk as the remaining ones turned into foes. My marital drama had reached my local Catholic Parish. My husband was excommunicated for marrying a second wife after marrying me in a white wedding. He later moved to another village where he bought a piece of land and settled there with his second family.

Due to the delays at the Nyanza General Hospital, I was referred to the Tenwek Hospital, where I was finally operated on after eight years. I stayed in the ward for three weeks without anyone, not even my husband, visiting me. My brother had financed the procedure. I had chosen not to involve Julian, because I did not want another round of anger-driven drama.

My faecal matter and blood clots stopped flowing after the surgery at Tenwek Hospital. But the urine did not stop flowing. The doctors referred me to Kenyatta National Hospital, but I did not have the funds to follow through.

I returned home, thanked my God for the little improvement I had had and adjusted myself psychologically to die wallowing in my pee. For four years, I lived with the mess. I watched as my thighs grew darker and darker due to the uric acid in the urine. I decided to continue going to church, now that there was no option.

It had been twelve years since I landed in my abyss. Twelve years-a-stinker! One afternoon, it was announced in church that a team of medics from Nairobi would be holding a medical camp at the Migori hospital for those suffering from fistula. Those with flowing urine and faeces were supposed to register with the hospital for the upcoming event. All heads in church shifted to my direction. This was when I realized that whatever I had been trying so hard to hide was an open secret. All these years, my struggles were as hidden as a cough!

I stood up, walked to the front and stood next to the official making the announcement. He stopped, gave me a disgusted stare and watched as a puddle of urine formed under the soles of my feet.

Noticing the awkward moment, the Italian priest stood up, walked to the front and picked the microphone. After clearing his voice, he said, "She is the shame of the village, isn't she? You may not say it, but I know how this village has been treating this woman."

Silence amid uncomfortable stares.

"There is this woman in the Bible who touched the hem of Jesus' garment. She got healed. While the woman in the Bible was bleeding, Angela Boke here is bleeding urine. She smells. She offends. And she is a shame. However, the reason that the medical camp is coming is her and the few others in your midst that you choose to hide and abuse in your homes…"

Everyone was attentive now.

"Whatever Angela is suffering from is very common. And the culture of circumcising your girls and marrying them off at a young age is one of the contributing factors to fistula. Angela will be treated, and you must assist her in this process."

He then turned to one of the altar boys and ordered for a basket. He placed it next to the offertory box and called out, "I need you to come forth."

Soon, members of the congregation lined up to put whatever they could in the basket. I stood there, mute. I had planned to take the microphone and insult everyone in that darn church. Thank heavens I was not allowed to speak.

Contributions done, the priest picked some notes from the basket and sent his driver to the shop. He later asked me to speak to him after the service. That day, I sat alone on a pew at the front, as the service proceeded. By the end of the mass, my urine was dripping on the floor, and formed a miniature stream.

After the mass, I went to the priest's office. He handed me a diaper and ordered me to go put it on in the toilet. I did. It felt very bulky but comfortable. When I returned, he handed me a brown envelope and ordered his driver to take me home – but not before reminding me to register for the medical camp.

Upon opening the envelope at home, I found 50,453 shillings ($504). The following morning, I went to the hospital and registered for the medical camp. I was not alone. There were other women from as far as Rongo, Homa Bay and other adjacent towns, also living with fistula. We were told to go back for screening and surgery after two weeks.

I then bought several diapers to last me a few more days and shopped for my household. For the first time in months, my children enjoyed sumptuous beef for supper.

I went to the health facility the following morning. I was the third person to be registered and screened. The medical staff told me to eat well since I was clearly unhealthy. The medic told me to stop worrying about people's epithets and eat well. After all, the urine would still flow, unless I was dead.

I went back home and embarked on the feeding programme. The more I ate, the heavier the flow was. However, I felt a sense of peace as I was being wheeled into the theatre. As the anaesthesia took effect, I recalled how I had arrived at the facility at almost 5:30 a.m. The medical team had arrived at around 8 a.m. They were taken around the facility, as a local member of staff took my essentials. She was struggling to maintain her calm due to my stench. Urine would well right under my buttocks before being absorbed by the diaper. No one accompanied me. My daughters knew where I was, but we had an agreement that they would keep this information to themselves.

My mind drifted back to Julian, his new family, and his new-found peace. His painful slaps, kicks and punches. I drifted into dreamland. To my childhood and my school days.

I woke up in a hospital ward at around at around 6 p.m., hungry and thirsty. A nurse walked over to me and asked me what I wanted. "I want anything edible," I answered. My mouth was dry. My palms felt as dry as wood with a stiff feeling around my waist. But my chest felt lighter. The nurse walked away and returned with a healthy meal on a platter. I cleared it in minutes. I then washed it down with two glasses of water.

I expected urine to start flowing, but nothing happened. I could not believe it. I sat down, and peeked at my groin. I was naked. As I bent over to check further, I felt a sharp pain in my belly. I let out a loud scream and slumped back in bed. The nurse rushed to my bedside.

"Don't do that. Don't strain. Just lie back and rest."

My previous normal was back. And it felt so abnormal! I realized that I was not alone. As I mulled over my new-found peace, a loud shriek filled the room. Damn! Some people can scream! I sat up, startled as the same pain cut through my inner belly. That was the moment I realized that I was not alone. The scream came from a patient who had just woken up and been welcomed by the searing pain. She could not stand it. The room was full of women. All sought to communicate in their native languages. Ekegusii, Kuria, Luo, Luhya and one from the so-called Kenyan Greek – Gikuyu.

"Wanjiru, it must have been tough dealing with the flow of poop and urine due to your people's love for flooded meals," one woman quipped. A short burst of laughter filled the room, before being filled with groans. They had strained their internal wounds. The people of the region are known for their love for copious amounts of soup in their meals.

"Food is never food without twenty litres of water, Irish potatoes and some carrots. I cannot accept an invitation without a confirmation of availability of soup!" Wanjiru fired back. No one laughed.

Two weeks later, and after days of exercise and other forms of therapy, I was discharged. My daughters had dutifully visited me in hospital every day, and were on call to take me back home. Julian's age mate and neighbour, who ran a taxi business at Kehancha, offered to take me home.

There, I found the house in a mess. Apparently, Julian had made an impromptu visit. And when he failed to find me, he concluded that I had eloped. He beat up my daughters and turned the house upside down. None of my daughters told him where I was. The girls rearranged the house as I waited outside. I slept on the couch since my bedding was charred by urine. The girls cleaned the house in the following days, and offered one of their mattresses and bedding for me. It was like a new wind was blowing in our house. The acrid smell reduced as days went by. I started regaining my health and colour. My blackened inner thighs started peeling and were later replaced by new skin. I was like a young girl down there.

My brother gave me 25,000 shillings ($ 250), with which I started a small grocery business at Kehancha. Word reached Julian that I was healed. He would pass by once in a while, and feign ignorance.

My business has since grown, and, thanks to the priest, I supply two local Catholic-run schools with greens. I have managed to spruce up my house, and even extend it.

Recently, two years after the surgery, my husband returned home. He claimed that he needed peace of mind. In the twelve years that I battled fistula, his first step-son had turned 20. The younger rascal was 18. The two boys were harassing their step-father, asking him to leave. They needed space. The mighty warrior is now aging, and cannot defend himself anymore. He had two children from the second marriage, both girls.

My daughters accepted their father back. I embraced him. He now stays with us, and retired after two years. He has since joined my business, and takes his time to educate his fellow men on the importance of supporting their spouse's fistula, stigma and any other medical issue.

My mother-in-law passed away a year ago, but had not made any effort to mend fences with us. Neither has Julian openly apologized. After all, the warrior in him still cannot allow his ego to stoop to a woman. He shows it through actions. Last month, his two daughters moved in with us. One suffers from mild cerebral palsy. I take care of them as mine. The other woman is banned from this house. In the trenches that lie between Ntimaru and Kegonge, more young men are still decimating each other just to own cows. The science that gave rise to guns that now kill us, is the same science that restored my health, and wealth.

Hail science!

Recovered and Rejoicing: Polly's Story

Motherhood is natural. Nothing beats being a mother. As mothers, we are vessels that connect the past, present and future generations.

My name is Polly Moraa. As my name indicates, I hail from Kisii County, where I was born and bred. Kisii is one of the counties that lie within the former Nyanza region. Its people are predominantly from the Bantu-speaking Abagusii tribe. The Abagusii people also neighbour Nyamira County, which was once part of Kisii. Apart from the Abagusii, the Kuria people of Migori County are also linguistically and anthropologically related to Abagusii. We are some of the few non-Nilotic communities that are natives of Nyanza. However, the Luo community, which is Nilotic, occupies a larger portion of Nyanza.

As a mother, nothing afflicts me more than losing a baby, be it during childbirth or even when the child is older.

I had returned to Kisii Teaching and Referral Hospital once again, lying on the bed as I waited for medics to take me through the all-familiar ritual, ahead of being wheeled into the theatre. As I waited, a feeling of déjà vu hit me. Not really déjà vu, but memories of a sickening experience that I would do anything to overcome. Grief, loss and engulfing desolation.

I saw a female figure walking towards my bed. Her steps were measured and graceful. She did not look like the abrasive medics that we are used to here. I sat up in anticipation.

"Okay, lady, how are you?"

"Fine, doctor."

"Yes, I am Doctor Valerie, I am here to see you today."

"I knew it. I immediately knew that you are not one of us. You are different," I said.

"I am not different. Actually, I am also from this Kisii region. It is just that I don't work here," she answered.

"Interesting, now why on earth don't you work here?" I asked her.

"We cannot all work here. Some of us must work at other facilities outside the region," she said, as she patted my shoulder, her face brightening into a wry smile.

Well, as I said earlier, my last visit here was not such a happy one.

I had been brought here after going into a difficult and prolonged labour. Upon being admitted, I watched in horror as medics pulled out my baby using forceps, with dark blood oozing from its bruises. That was not normal at all. I had given birth before and never seen metallic objects being used to tug at an infant. That grimly puzzled and filled me with fear. Doctors later on informed me that my baby was dead.

From then on, my leakages escalated.

I cannot recall what happened, but ever since I was a young girl, I used to have a problem holding my urine. I would often rush to the toilet immediately I felt like passing urine or else, I would end up soiling my poor self.

When I met my husband for the first time, I was open to him about it. He was very understanding and stood by me for the twenty-two years that we lived together. He even decided to keep it away from his parents and relatives. This protected me from ridicule and possible bullying from my in-laws. Unfortunately, he passed away recently from a liver disease. He had been hooked to cheap liquor and would often fall critically ill, necessitating admission. Doctors had warned him against taking acidic foods and alcohol. The advice fell on deaf ears.

For years, I was forced to take up the breadwinner's role. In a region that is known to be relatively conservative, I think my husband was one among very few men who appreciated their wives and the women in their lives. Even with his weaknesses, his death robbed me of a wonderful companion. He was human, after all.

Now, as I lay there, engaging this doctor, I could still feel a huge sense of loss. The loss of my baby, my husband and my self-esteem. The uncontrolled flow of body fluids had been my biggest challenge. While I had my issue with bladder control, I never experienced such nasty flow of stool. I never smelt so bad. Never had I felt people's nasty looks stab me so hard. It was extremely distressing.

I had gone to the health facility a few days earlier, after being informed that some doctors from Nairobi would be performing surgeries on patients with problems similar to mine free of charge. Dr Sabina happened to be one of them.

"Did you seek any help from your relatives?" she asked.

"No. It would have been tricky for me. Look, my father is polygamous. With wives and my siblings to deal with, I saw no need to bother him. He is also old and sickly."

This condition had made it hard for me to interact with my colleagues at the market. Look, I am a small-scale trader at a local market. My work entails hauling heavy loads. I was doing it, but lately, I noticed that customers have been keeping away from my stall, because I stunk more than a skunk. Some of the snoots at the market even used my unfortunate case to bad-mouth me. They said that I was not hygienic enough to handle food. So bad was the situation that lately, I had stopped going there. I now stayed at home, begging for alms. The habit of depending on handouts had never defined my life at all.

"You will be fine after this surgery, God willing," Dr Sabina said reassuringly. "How long were you in labour before arriving here?"

"I had stayed for several hours after my water broke. I live far away from here and we don't have health facilities around," I answered.

"That prolonged labour raptured parts of your bladder and rectal muscles, which messed up your bowel movement," she concluded and walked away.

It was actually after that failed delivery, three years ago, that I started having this problem. I recall how my relatives, led by my father-in-law, came to the hospital and picked the infant's body for burial at home. I was left there for days. The baby I never saw nor held was interred in my absence. That was the baby I never bonded with as a mother. I should have been allowed to set my eyes on the baby's corpse for closure. I still mourn my baby. I feel like they lied to me.

I heard that the body was buried in a carton. That is how it is done in many Kenyan communities. A child with no name and no physical relation. The baby that was known to have existed in me, but not beyond. I still miss my baby, yet it feels so odd that I do.... I was later shown the little grave where they buried it. It had sunk. Nature was in the process of reclaiming its space.

As thoughts clouded my mind, my eyes trained on the white ceiling, I was wheeled into a room and then, darkness.

I woke up in a ward. There were several of us. Some women from as far as Nyamira, Kisumu and even Kakamega were there. They had all just been operated on. I understood that our bills were fully covered. I am forever grateful to those who made it possible for us to be attended to.

Suddenly, I felt some slight pain in my belly. "I can handle that," I assured myself. It was a welcome pain. With the operation, the doctors had accorded me and my fellow women a dignified life. A life free from shame.

Two weeks later, I was discharged. However, I was ordered to continue with the exercises that we had been undertaking since the surgical procedures. They were meant to facilitate the healing process. After a month, I went back to my market stall. However, someone else had since occupied it. As we argued over it, one of my former colleagues who still ran a business there joined in. Baba Kelvin was a burly man with an authoritative voice.

"Young man, I'm sure you were informed that that stall belonged to a lady who fell sick. Go get your refund from whoever leased it to you and get out of here. The owner is back!" he snarled.

"But I understand that she pees and poops on herself. That is why she left. She cannot handle food for human consumption. Too dirty," he fired back.

"She is all right now. She was treated recently," Baba Kelvin answered.

"When did we start treating curses?" He was getting into my hair now.

More and more traders gathered around as the argument went south.

"Young man, this is not a curse," I responded.

"You think we don't know? You are one of those women who were bewitched by their husbands and in-laws for selling their bodies. Can you go back to where you came from? You are not cut out for this business." I felt like smashing his nose. Now, that hurt. I sat down and started crying.

"Have you ever been a woman? Do you have a womb? Do you experience monthly periods?" I shouted at the boy angrily. Everyone else kept quiet.

"What I had had nothing to do with curses or witchcraft. It was caused by prolonged labour. It is called fistula. Stop acting ignorant. It can befall anyone," I said. People were keenly listening.

"But I am not moving. This is my stall. Take your fistula and go away!" the kid stubbornly said.

Baba Kelvin now got agitated and moved towards the young man. More and more male traders joined him. They began roughing up the lad.

"Okay! Okay!" he shouted. "Let me sell today and move out tomorrow."

"No. Get out now. Go sell your wares where you came from. We don't want a mannerless young fellow like you running your dirty mouth here. You have been a pain in the neck since you invited yourself here," Baba Kevin bellowed.

The cowed young chap gathered his stuff and left, but not without throwing me an epithet about my womanhood.

"If what came out of his backside was as much as what came out of his filthy mouth, we would all be covered in his waste here," one trader shouted as the lad walked away, his sack swinging off his shoulder.

The young trader was not alone. Many have shaped opinion about me and my health issue.

My colleagues milled around me, some secretly sniffing me. I did not smell of faecal matter. I reeked no urine. I was a new Pauline. Days later, I was back to the market, buying and selling goods. Out of curiosity, some clients streamed back, to buy and to enquire, growing my earnings in the process. My future now looked hopeful for myself and my family.

A month later, Mama Levin whispered to me, "I need your advice." She was one of the sellers who often sneered at me and spoke ill about me with the aim of winning my clients. "Look ... my fourteen-year-old daughter might be having the problem you had. I don't know where to take her."

I stared at her. At fourteen years, how did the girl end up with a fistula?

"You know what kids have become nowadays. The internet and the penetration of smartphones are exposing them to inappropriate stuff. She has been playing around with boys. She became pregnant. She cannot tell who is responsible for the pregnancy. She was due last week. We took her to our local clinic, but she unfortunately lost the baby.

When they discharged her, we noticed that urine was coming out involuntarily. That was shocking."

I advised Mama Levin to take her to the Kisii Teaching and Referral Hospital immediately. I hope she did.

I am a Queen Rising from my Foulness

At the tender, yet mature age of twenty-two, Beatrice Nkasiogi radiates love and an air of felicity. Her native name means 'the one who is always in hurry'.

Standing tall a few inches shy of six feet, her looks betray her Nilo-Cushitic Maasai ancestry. Her bewitching beauty, capped by her laid-back demeanor seals her place in the pavilions of beauty. In her native Kibiku area of Kenya's Kajiado County, she is viewed by her peers as a daughter of the soil. She oozes nativity and sophistication.

Kajiado County flanks Kenya's capital, Nairobi, to the north – and sprawls all the way to the south, sharing a shoulder with the neighbouring Tanzania. The Masaai people are considered custodians of wildlife in the East African region. It is a position that has seen them rise to an iconic position in the global realm of tourism. The county's pride is the Amboseli National Park that also boasts of the big five and other animal species.

Although the Masaai people are considered natives of Kajiado and Narok, they are also found in Laikipia County. They also have cousins in Samburu, Turkana and Ilchamus tribes, also found in the expansive Rift Valley region. There is also a substantive population of the Masaai people in the neighbouring Tanzania. All these tribes fall under a family called the Maa-speaking community.

Like a beautiful rose that carries a painful spike beneath its stem, the Maasai culture has its own dark side that perils women. For example, it allows men to marry girls as young as nine years. There is also a custom called beading, which allows young warriors – called Morans – to sleep with young girls whom they are not obligated to marry.

Back to Beatrice… although her parents hail from Kajiado, they worked in Narok County, which is over 250 kilometres away. For this, she grew up in both counties and would visit her native home in Kajiado during the holidays.

As they say, when we have no trouble, trouble comes looking for us. But until it happened, little did this lady know that her bewitching beauty could also rob her of the joys of her youth.

One evening, while still in primary school, she met a dashing young man who stole her young heart. Love was one of the many things that she was discovering and exploring as she turned fourteen. But it was blissful only while it lasted. With gifts and sweet words and all manner of flattering tricks, the brash chap tricked her into early sex. Hers was one of the many perils that line the paths of young girls in Kenya and sub-Saharan Africa.

Furthermore, she had also seen her friends engage in the act, with some classmates getting married after undergoing female circumcision – a practice that is still rampant in the Masaai community. She never thought she could fall pregnant, until it happened.

"I tried to keep it under wraps for some months," she quips. But mothers being mothers, her little secret would soon come to be a secret no more.

"One day, my mother called me and demanded to know who was responsible. I was lost for words… I mean, how could she notice it so easily?" she asks defeatedly.

"Well, I had already informed Ben, my then boyfriend, that I was carrying his baby. He made promises to marry me, but later cut off communication. He dissolved into thin air. He switched off his mobile phone and later moved out of Narok town. It was very hard for me to trace him. The fool disappeared… I have never felt so abandoned. I later heard that he was married and had moved back to his village. He had three wives already. I had a very difficult conversation with mum, who later allowed me to keep my baby, but immediately took me to a local clinic for antenatal care," she adds sardonically.

Her mother allowed her to continue with her education until she was six months into her pregnancy. That was when she relocated back to her rural home in Kajiado. Unfortunately, she left behind her maternal care booklet in Narok. Back home in Kajiado, Beatrice moved in with her aunt because there was no one at home to take care of her.

"I just stayed at home doing domestic chores as my aunt watched over me. I was not attending school at all," she quips.

In her seventh month of pregnancy, Beatrice sought antenatal services at a local clinic.

"I was turned away because I did not have the booklet. The medical workers told me that I could not be attended to without the initial booklet."

She returned to the hospital one week later, armed with a new booklet. However, she was once again turned away, as the hospital staff demanded the old booklet with her initial records from Narok. Dejected and lost, the then little girl returned to her aunt's home and resigned to fate.

She continued with the usual domestic chores as her aunt watched over her, unknown to them that the delivery day was nigh.

"One morning, I was busy doing the dishes when I felt some liquid run down my thighs, to my ankles and to the floor. I screamed. My aunt rushed into the kitchen, took one look at me and told me that my water had broken. It was a surreal experience. I mean, it was totally unexpected. I was not in any pain. It was very puzzling, hence my disbelief. I just stayed there as my aunt instructed me to wait for labour pain."

Two days later, pain descended.

The more she held on, the more the pain heightened. It reached a point when she could not hold any more. Her clenched teeth gave way to cries, then wails. It was at that moment that her aunt took her to a nearby hospital on the third day. By the time they arrived at the private hospital, Beatrice was in so much pain that she passed out. When she came to, she found herself at the Kajiado Referral Hospital, where the doctors informed her that she had lost her baby. The baby had died in the uterus.

"I was crushed. I mean, I had not seen the baby. I still don't know its gender. I should have been allowed to hold the baby's corpse just for a second. To see its features … for closure."

As she lay on her bed, mired by thoughts of grief over her lost baby, nurses cleaning her were talking. One of them mentioned to her colleague that something was leaking.

Upon shifting and turning, she realized that she had soiled herself. Urine mixed with faeces. Now that was strange!

"I just couldn't understand how both came out without my knowledge. I was too weak to even think, but this really disturbed me."

Beatrice stayed in hospital for almost two weeks, and was later transferred to the Kenyatta National Hospital. The hospital is the oldest referral facility in Kenya, and serves the Eastern African region as well.

She stayed in admission for over two months, as her parents struggled with medical bills. She was discharged after the then serving Nairobi Governor, who, offered to offset her bills. She was one of the beneficiaries of the politician's philanthropic acts, which often drew mixed reactions in the political scene. Sonko had run a populist campaign in the 2017 elections and won by a landslide. However, he later lost his seat as the intricate political intrigues of Kenya swallowed its children.

Upon heading home from hospital, Beatrice later joined her parents in Narok, where she returned to school, but with a repellent condition. She had no control over her bowels.

"I still could not understand why urine and poop would roll down my thighs and into my shoes. The stench was too nauseating, unsettling and repulsive to bear. Doctors recommended adult diapers. And they are not cheap," she says.

At home, neither her parents nor her siblings discussed her condition. However, her schoolmates did. Some accused her of having wronged her ancestors. Others blamed her for being of loose morals and having had sex with adults who raptured her reproductive organs.

"Some boys would even refer to me as 'that loose girl who stinks'. Those were very hurtful epithets."

Every morning, her mother would hand her a diaper for the day. She needed two diapers per day. She would head home from her nearby school to change and return for the afternoon classes.

"Sometimes, the urine and poop would be too much, causing the diaper to leak. Diapers would sit very uncomfortably between my thighs, making me walk with an ugly gait. I would sometimes run out of class during sessions, as soon as I saw my classmates start fanning their noses. I watched as my parents struggled to purchase diapers. Each adult diaper costs around 150 Kenya Shillings ($ 1.50). Soon, my father requested for help from our church. Congregants would later chip in," she says.

One day, her father returned from work with news.

"Kenyatta National Hospital was asking for people with my condition to go for screening. AMREF would cater for the costs of reconstructive surgeries for the lucky ones," she reveals.

Two weeks later, Beatrice and her father walked into Kenyatta National Hospital. She was not alone. There, she met with women of varied creeds, ages and tribes, all battling uncontrollable bowel movement.

"When my turn came, I sat opposite a female doctor, who calmly introduced herself to me as Dr Sabina. I was taken by her laid-back mien. Deep inside, I wondered how she was able to withstand the stench emitted by us," she says.

"This is when I decided to ask her what I was suffering from. She coolly took a piece of paper and drew circles, explaining the workings of a female reproductive system. She explained that when my water broke, the baby was still hanging somewhere up in my pelvis. Therefore, the baby was far. This prolonged my labour. It resulted in the foetus sitting on my muscles for long, thus piling pressure on the bladder and causing the urine to leak. She also explained that the process of delivery was determined by the birth canal, size of the baby, the mother's age, psyche and strength, together with the strength of contractions. In my case, the lack of antenatal records also complicated matters for the medical teams."

Beatrice, like many of her fellow patients, was operated on and later discharged after two weeks. Her parents never incurred any costs. African Medical and Research Foundation, as promised, footed the bill.

"Every morning, Dr Khisa, who had performed the operation, would pass by my bed and reassure me of total healing. God works through humans like Dr Khisa and Sabina," Beatrice adds.

Every day she walks into the toilet, she appreciates the efficacy of the surgery.

"Every day, my mother's eyes would well with tears as she handed me yet another diaper. My father's face was always filled with nothing but despondency. Now, I see a sheen of hope in my parents, who continue standing with me as I rebuild my self-esteem that was battered by years of shame and derision. I am a queen rising from my foulness."

Beatrice has completed her secondary school education, and is now expecting to join college soon. As she looks back at her times with fistula, she draws her lessons and lives in her present joy, as she thanks those who gave her a reason to smile. She specifically thanks her parents for standing with her during her dark moment. Those were truly her defining days, when times were bad.

$Part_2$

Stories narrated by family members

Perspectives of Family Members on Obstetric Fistula

Background

Fistula has a far-reaching effect on the family members of the affected women. It drives husbands, family and friends away, because in the first place, they do not understand this new condition that the woman in their lives finds herself in. This, coupled with the possible stillbirth of the child they had been waiting for, does not make matters easier.

Family members in particular and the community in general should therefore take charge and lead the way in ensuring that women with fistula get the required financial and psychological help that they need. They also need to show understanding of this situation that these women find themselves in. It is enough that they suddenly have to deal with embarrassing leakages and loss of their children; dealing with societal stigma magnifies this desperate situation that the women find themselves in.

However, if more awareness was created at the family level, then family members would be able to support women dealing with fistula, easing their fistula burden and also help them get the necessary treatment, so that they can start living a normal life, just like they did before. In addition to financial help, what these women need is understanding and acceptance from the family and society. The family therefore needs to make a conscious choice to protect, support and defend their rights.

Casual Emergency!

I could not stomach the sight of my wife sprawling on the floor, writhing in pain and howling insults at me, apparently for impregnating her and therefore surrendering her to agony. It had been forty hours of labour, part of it spent on hoping that somehow the skilful hands of the midwife would resolve the suffering that had visited my wife. The last ten hours of the forty were distributed between doing anything and everything to get the baby out.

"Push! Push!" we screamed at Selina, my wife.

"I am pushing," she kept affirming amidst groans, grunts and grumbles.

"Push harder! That's the trick… harder!" the midwife advised, to which Selina would respond by insulting me, and twice or thrice our unborn child.

Every minute, hope diminished. We had all depended on the knowledge and skills of the midwife but looking at her face then, you could see worry written all over it. Finally, she appeared to throw in the towel. She stopped everything she was doing, which sent the signal for all of us to do the same, given that all actions in that small hut were based on her directives.

"What next?" Selina's mother asked the question that was running in everyone's mind.

"It's the child," said the midwife confidently.

"What about my child?" I jumped in defensively.

"He takes after you. He has a big head," the midwife cut in.

"So what?"

"We cut her open, that's what we do. The head cannot go through."

In that moment, the only sounds in the room were Selina's weeping, wailing and whimpers. That was for a moment, before the midwife spoke again. "The men will have to get out," she demanded. No reason was given.

There were six of us in that room: Selina's mother, Selina's sister, my mother, the midwife, Selina and myself, which meant that I was 'the men' she was referring to. I protested, but she promptly assumed command.

"The men must get out," she insisted.

"Why?" my mother came to my defence.

The midwife instantly turned our attention to Selina again. In between her, we could see a foreign body emerging. "There is your little man; he is coming out," the midwife said in a calm voice.

Immediately, it dawned on me that there were two men in the room and indeed both needed to get out. My little man was stuck on his way out and help was in the hands of the midwife. As for me, it was a question of tradition. The birth of a child is sacrosanct and a man must be as far away as possible from the process, lest he risks a curse to the unborn. That is what tradition dictates. I gave in.

I closed my eyes and walked out. The door to the hut was locked behind me. I began walking farther and farther away until I could no longer hear Selina's voice. Little did I realize that my son had lost a lot of blood during the cutting! A mother's instinct was at work, that was why Selina was crying, she did not hear her baby cry as she pushed that final lap.

Nevertheless, the wait was long. Minutes and more minutes passed as I waited. I felt the temptation to burst back into the hut and be part of the happenings. A train of thoughts filled my mind. I was both anxious and scared. I fidgeted, I walked around, I sweated, and certainly my body was not spared too from shivering. Generally, I was unsettled.

When the door of the hut was opened, I bolted back.

"Get the bicycle now!" Selina's mother directed.

I did not ask any question or seek any explanation. We had thought through this and I had prepared the bicycle, even washed it, in case of an emergency. Quickly, I went to our main house where I had kept it.

It was missing. I panicked.

"Where is my bicycle?" I shouted loud enough to get answers from anyone who could hear.

"Obed has gone with it to the *posho* mill just now," an answer followed; I could not tell from whom … perhaps the casual labourers digging in the farm, perhaps a passerby… someone. Obed took care of our cows at home.

My mind registered the problem, but it was not the time to grumble. I sped to the kitchen and picked a wheelbarrow.

Selina was helped into the wheelbarrow. We raced up a few hills, down as many valleys and through narrow paths and thickets, and anywhere there was a shortcut. The nearest hospital was ten kilometres away. What saved us was an old jalopy, a pickup truck belonging to the headteacher of a local school who stopped to give us a lift. His was one of the three vehicles in our locality. It was luck that brought him to us, however, that was not for long.

After about five kilometres, the vehicle came to a halt. The fuel tank had been emptied by the short journey. We divided responsibilities amongst ourselves. Seeing as we had left the wheelbarrow behind, I would carry Selina and together with the midwife and Selina's sister, we would pace towards the hospital. Selina's mother and my mother would guard the vehicle as the headteacher ran with a container to the nearest petrol station to look for fuel. The idea was that they would eventually catch up with us after the vehicle was refuelled. They never did! What happened, as I later learnt, was that after refuelling, they realized that the vehicle had other substantial problems that required it to be pushed back home and wait for when the headteacher could afford the services of a mechanic.

We arrived at the hospital exhausted to the limit, thanks to a second bout of luck in the form of a police car that once again gave us a lift.

There was a long queue at the hospital when we arrived. Everyone was looking sicker than the next person and every attempt to jump the queue was resisted by contemptuous stares. There was no healthcare worker with a free hand to assess the different levels of emergency and assist those that needed urgent help. The place was like a marketplace.

As we were still convincing some of the patients that we had in our hands the bigger problem, a nurse walked towards us rather casually.

"Pregnant woman, move here!" she instructed, directing us to a room at the end of the hallway. I had imagined that perhaps a stretcher would be available for this kind of situation, which did not turn out to be the case. My wife was admitted in this very room where other women were crying due to labour pains. Others had just escorted friends and family while others like us were lost for words and direction. My thought process was lost, the fact that my wife was badly cut in the process of childbirth gave me chills. She was oozing both blood and faecal matter with no sign of stopping. It was very confusing. How I wished that it was a bad dream but I was wrong; she had a big problem to deal with in an environment that was nothing close to private. My mind raced. Where else could we get help? I wondered what would happen to my son, not knowing he had passed on either during birth or shortly thereafter.

As fate would have it, almost six hours after we had arrived, the same nurse walked back to the waiting room at 6 p.m. We were still hurdled in the same room, patients and relatives interacted freely. Obed had joined us, with the bicycle, to take charge of the transportation of our new family member back home. In between the waiting hours, we had been furnished with information that the surgery conducted by the midwife back home had failed. She had sliced a piece of the child's head and cut up a few wrong places which she failed to stitch properly, thus resolving the situation in the hospital theatre would take some time. Part of the reason we were given was the fact that the only doctor who could carry out the procedure had gone to another facility to attend to other patients. All these explanations were just to pass time because my son was already dead by the time we arrived at the hospital.

"You will have to come back tomorrow but your wife will stay here," the nurse said.

"Why?" we responded in an imperfect chorus.

She explained that Selina was asleep, recovering from the surgery that was done to close the hole that had developed during childbirth. The abnormal communication had occurred between the rectum and birth canal, leading to oozing of faecal matter and urine.

"Then we will wait," my mother said.

"We don't have a bedroom in this hospital," the nurse retorted.

"We don't need a bedroom. There is enough space around here; we will stand if we have to," Selina's mother countered.

"All right," was all the nurse said before disappearing.

For the ten hours, we did not see her again. Any other nurse was of no help because somehow, we could only access information from the nurse who handled us first, unless a handover was done. After all, the hospital was too full, and you would be an idiot to expect that any nurse would have some free time on their hands.

"So, you are still here?" the nurse asked us the following morning when she arrived.

We did not have the energy to exchange words. All we could do was ask how Selina and the baby were.

"Wait here," she said and left.

We did not see her for another three hours. The anxiety and stress levels were rising by the moment. Selina's mother was hypertensive, which made things even harder for me. What could I do but wait and keep waiting?

We later caught up with the nurse in the corridors as she was passing by.

"Oh! Your case," she remarked, almost in a surprised tone.

"Come," she said.

We walked with her to the maternity wing of the hospital. She made us wait for her outside before rejoining us a few minutes later.

"Follow me," she signalled us.

We walked behind her one hallway after another, one pavement after another and one foyer after another. Finally, at the end of one of the hallways, we went down a staircase to the basement of the building. The environment was cold and filled with whirring sounds.

When we walked in, I realized that I was all alone with the nurse. My mother, Obed, Selina's mother and sister, remained at the entrance. I did not know why but whom could I ask? I maintained my silence. Little did I know that they had seen the writing on the door, which I had missed. The nurse took me to the morgue, handed me to the attendant and just walked away. It took time for me to realize that we were in a morgue. The attendant was still writing some details in the register. He said nothing at that moment.

"Wait, what's going on?" I asked.

"I have been told that you are the one who brought the new mother yesterday," the mortician said.

"Yes, but why are we in a mortuary?" I shot back, my heart beating audibly.

"To view the body of course," he responded.

"Whose body? What happened to my wife?"

He simply pulled the fridge open. I almost puked. I had never in my life seen the lifeless body of an infant. That was my first time, and it was my child, my own son – the heir to my inheritance.

The rest of the family had joined me by this time. The mood was sombre. Shock stood in the place of tears. Obed almost fainted. Calmly, Selina's mother asked to be shown where her daughter was. It was the kind of calm that was a time bomb, which made the request one that you could not turn down.

The mortician asked us to wait there as he went ahead to look for the nurse.

"While I am gone, please do not receive any fresh corpses on my behalf," he said walking out of the door, as though it was a possibility or the norm.

When the nurse arrived, I could not hold myself together.

"When did this happen and why didn't you tell us?" I yelled at her.

"People die and children die too. We cannot resurrect them!" she responded.

Really? Was it too hard to just tell me that my son was no more? That he had lost a lot of blood during birth and the travel to hospital took time?

The emergency was handled poorly because the doctor also took too long to come to the hospital and attend to my son. Did they just commit a malpractice, negligence or was it the norm? Why were they so heartless? Why me? I lamented silently.

Selina was still asleep after the operation to repair the rectal fistula. When we arrived at the ward where she had been assigned, we were confused because the room was not conducive for immediate post-operative care. It was a general ward, a hall designed like a ballroom with beds lined up from one end to the other. It was a chaotic environment with newborn babies crying and laughing, mothers chatting with each other, visiting friends and relatives walking up and down. There was an overall sense of disorder.

Selina's bed was stationed right in the symmetrical middle of the room where she was surrounded by this anarchy. She was excited when she woke up to see us surrounding her bed. I held her hand firmly.

Does she know? I asked myself. We all seemed to ask ourselves the same question. No one was courageous enough to bring it up. It was almost as if we had entered into a conspiracy of silence, whose end goal was to wait for cues from her. It did not take long.

"I knew you wanted a son," Selina told me. "The nurse told me it's a boy," she added.

We looked at each other in silence.

"I think we can name him after your late father, what do you think?" Selina continued to speak. I did not respond.

"Come on," she urged me on. I did not respond again.

What I hated most in that short period of time was the idea that the heavy burden of breaking the news of the lifelessness of our son had been squarely placed on my shoulders. By whom? I did not know; I could not guess. For that reason, I did not even know where to start. I excused myself and left my mother to tell her the whole truth and nothing but the truth. I could not handle it. I was lost for words. The realization that she had a bad rectal tear, lost her baby and nobody said a thing was just too much to bear. I just left.

Walking into town, I found a bar and drowned in the beer. What else could I do? Maybe if the nurse had broken the news differently or at least prepared me and my mother or mother-in-law or the larger family on how to handle Selina after surgery, things would have been different.

At times I blame myself. Looking back, I see gaps during the home birth. I should have insisted on staying in the hut to see my son, feel him, hold and embrace him and create some connection with him. It just did not occur to me that he would soon die, even before I could name him after my father as is the tradition. As a friend once said, "Your wife is alive Jeff, soon you will be blessed with another baby." Maybe he was right, maybe he was not – because there are no two people who are alike in any family and no child can replace another one.

What I am grateful for is that Selina had immediate surgery to repair the fistula so she did not experience the ridicule and stigma associated with the condition. As they say, experience is the best teacher. Next time, no traditional midwife will touch my wife. As soon as labour begins, I will take her to a hospital to give birth, a place where midwives and doctors are responsive and compassionate. I indeed learnt my lessons.

Worlds Apart

I was not going to bathe with that cold water, I vowed. The weather had been unrepentantly cold in the last two days and it had threatened my relationship with water. Schools were closed and there were no weddings to attend. Torturing my body with freezing water while there was no special event was very unwise. I considered myself a very wise person and I also knew that a wise person bathes only when necessary. Therefore, I decided that I would only surrender my face, part of my hands and legs to the cold baptism.

"Ekeko!" I heard Uncle Obaga shout as he pushed the noisy wooden gate open. I hastily abandoned my bathing trials and ran to where he was. I did not understand why he always called me Ekeko while my name was Edwin. Why he also preferred shouting to talking calmly like his peers baffled me. A young girl of about fifteen years, my age, followed him shyly. She had a tiny, rugged backpack tightly squeezed under her right armpit. Her clothes were old and her skin seemed like it had not interacted with water or oil for several weeks. But she had a beautiful round face with pointed breasts.

"This is your new aunty, she is called Waridi. Show her around," Uncle Obaga blurted while belching violently. How could I call my age mate Aunty? What was wrong with Uncle? I wanted to protest but I swallowed my words and humbly replied, "Yes Uncle."

Since I came into Uncle Obaga's house, he had chased away three 'aunties'. The last one had left a week before because she forgot to put enough salt in Uncle's potatoes. Uncle had thrown her out in the night. It was raining heavily. He asked her to go back to her mother to learn how to put salt in food.

Waridi was shy and had a rather deep voice that was not particularly feminine. We did not talk much. The torn bag she wrapped under her armpit concealed a few things which I figured to be clothes and a small diary. I showed her where to get firewood, where to fetch water, where to wash clothes from among other places that a woman needed to be shown. After the short orientation, Uncle called her into his room and closed the door. Uncle had always done this with the aunties.

They would always scream. But Waridi's scream was different. It had undertones of pain; I could feel it. Poor girl.

It was months after we had resumed school but Waridi never went to school with us. She had revealed to me that her parents had married her off to Uncle with the promise that he would school her and help her grow. However, the only thing that Uncle helped Waridi grow was her stomach. It was increasing in size every day.

One time as we were harvesting maize, Waridi lay down and started to cry in pain. I rushed to her but she would not let me touch her. Even so, I did not know what to do. What was I to do with a pregnant woman who did not want any help? Uncle was away at Mamoto's Liquor Joint, his favourite place to shed the week's stress off. He particularly loved to go there during the morning hours and never wanted anybody to disturb him while he took his alcohol. At one time, my class teacher had paid us a visit to inquire why he had not paid my school fees. He was not at home. I had to look for him at the drinking den. He was so furious that he slapped me twice and asked me to tell that teacher to mind his own business.

"I will pay when I will pay!" he shouted after me.

Perhaps that was why as I went to fetch him, I was afraid that he would slap me again for interrupting his happy moments. But this was a life-and-death matter. Aunty was with child and in pain. I missed him at Mamoto's Liquor Joint and traversed five of his favourite dens, but he was nowhere to be found. In each of the dens, the patrons reported not to have seen him for a long time. He was heavily in debt hence might have gone in search of new joints where he was not known. I gave up the search and decided to run back home to Aunty. Maybe my presence would be of more help than the hopeless search for her husband.

But Aunty Waridi was not at home. I became afraid. I became confused. What might have happened to her? And where might she have gone to? She was not in the banana plantations nor was she in Uncle's room. Maybe Uncle had come home while I was looking for him and taken her to hospital. I sighed and continued with the maize harvesting. I kept praying that she delivers safely, and twins too. Her stomach was very big. It had to be twins.

When Uncle crawled into the compound three hours later, dead drunk and shouting for Waridi to make him soup, I was terrified. Where was Waridi? I related to the drunkard the events surrounding Waridi but he did not seem to care. All he wanted was soup. Hot soup and silence, thereafter, he wanted to sleep. I had to prepare him his soup and as he snored like a malfunctioned automobile afterwards, I sneaked out to ask in the neighbourhood about Waridi's whereabouts. Nobody had any information. Nobody said anything helpful.

It was on a Wednesday, three days after pregnant Waridi disappeared. I had just come back from school and was busy preparing a meal for Uncle. I watched Waridi struggle to open the short wooden gate and ran to help her. She was not carrying a child, but her stomach was still big. Maybe she had not yet delivered. She looked tired and sad. Her smile was equally tired and forced. In the silence and short distance that we walked to the house, I realized that her walking style was also different. Where was she from and where were the twins? I pondered, but was afraid to ask her. Her face did not welcome any question. I also rarely talked to her when Uncle was around, unless in whispers.

She had barely settled before Uncle pounced on her.

"Where have you been, you fool?" Uncle demanded while pushing her to the wall.

I felt sorry for her. She began to narrate how she struggled to the hospital where she lost her baby. It crushed me. It disturbed me more when I observed her face. It was tired but not helplessly mournful. She was either too shocked to mourn or the situation had sapped all the energy in her. I was afraid to look at her. For the first time, I witnessed Uncle lack words to shout. He was equally shocked but not particularly remorseful.

"Who took you to the hospital?" he asked again.

Waridi was quiet, she was not listening. She was lost in her own dark thoughts. Secretly mourning perhaps or silently nursing her pain. The following morning, I heard Uncle shout in anger and disgust.

"A mature woman wetting the bed like a foolish child! Who birthed you idiot?"

As much as I did not agree with Uncle's last sentiment, I also privately wondered how a grown-up girl could urinate on the bed.

I failed to understand. I, however, felt sorry for her. The pain of losing her child must have clouded her mind.

In the weeks and months that followed, Aunty was always wetting herself without thought. Uncle would slap her each time and even chased her out of the house at night.

"Rubbish!" Uncle would shout after her.

I had also started to avoid Aunty Waridi because of her awful smell. It was really terrible. Uncle's permanent drunkenness always seemed to block his huge nose from smelling the odour. But any time that he did, he would quarrel her for farting around him without shame. Waridi's protests that she was not the one who did it only earned her slaps and unthinkable abuses. I knew it was not fart, for that bad smell was permanently with her after she came from the hospital. It is as if she left her senses there. Why could she not clean herself and control her bladder? I pitied her but I was also angry at her. Why would anyone be named after a fresh flower (*waridi* is Swahili for rose) which smelt pleasant, only for the person to smell like the rotten version of the flower?

It was on a Sunday. Uncle's friends had paid us a visit. Each time Waridi went to where they were to refill their liquor and food, many would hold their noses and complain of an awful smell. They looked at her suspiciously. Emali, Uncle's best friend was the first to react verbally. Emali was always loud, just like Uncle. He spoke a lot but nothing sensible, though he always thought of himself as very wise.

"Your wife smells like a rotten rat, where did you find this one this time?" he asked as he indifferently sipped his liquor.

The others laughed out aloud in their drunken states. Uncle was ashamed but chose not to talk. He too laughed, but reluctantly, not with his usual energy. It was not long after that Waridi walked back to refill the drinking pots of the guzzlers, afraid and nursing a mountain of shame. She had heard Emali talk about her. But it was never going to be the same again. As she rose from the pots, urine loosely came down her thighs, wetting her dress. I was so ashamed that I chose to look away.

"This one is bewitched brother. You married a curse," Emali chimed in again.

I did not want to witness what would transpire afterwards. The humiliation was overwhelming. Uncle would never recover from it. I disappeared and went away until evening after they had left. That night, Uncle beat her senseless. She had to sleep outside because Uncle did not want a stinking wife beside him. But Waridi was never a big crier. She never let out a loud cry. Only tears would come down her face.

When she wetted herself again the following day, Uncle decided that he had had enough. I had never seen anyone so angry! He literally dragged Waridi out of the house and asked her to go back to her parents.

"What is this I married?" he regretted loudly.

I was even afraid he would also throw me out. I feared for Waridi, where would she go at that time of the night alone? I wanted to beg Uncle to allow her spend the night and leave the following morning but he was never a man to be questioned or advised by children. He would have asked me to follow her. And where would I go, I had no other home.

I feared for what might befall her. The last time she disappeared, and in pain, she lost her child. My memory of her was always burdened with unnamed fear. I prayed for her constantly. After she left, Uncle never mentioned her again, ever.

I never saw or heard about Waridi for a long time. Another aunty replaced her and my uncle's life moved on. We soon forgot about her until one day when I was at the hospital battling malaria. I felt someone tap my shoulders. I looked behind. At first, I could not place her face, then something about her smile struck. It was Waridi! She had another man by her side. I would not have recognized her if she had not reached out. It was hard to identify her. She had grown and changed. Her face though still beautiful, was laden with old sadness. A sadness that was borne of years of pain and loss. I was curious to know what had happened to her over the years and where she had gone. Waridi, as if reading my mind and my unspoken thoughts, was willing to relate her story to me. First, she joyfully introduced the man beside her as her loving husband. Unlike Uncle Obaga, he was not loud and he did not shout.

"I am here for a fistula checkup," Waridi mentioned.

I was lost, I had never heard of that part of the body. My biology classes must have gone to waste. Fearing that I sounded ignorant, I responded that I was equally there for the same. Together with her husband, they burst out laughing. They noticed my arrogant ignorance. She then sat me down to narrate how her first pregnancy with Uncle Obaga had caused her fistula and the loss of their child. When she left that night, she found her way to her brother's house where she lived for three years before meeting Tommy, her husband.

As she narrated her story, I felt guilty, I felt ashamed. While I was angry at her for being careless with her bladder and not bathing, she was suffering from an unknown ailment that she had no control over. All she needed was medical help.

"I came back that day since nobody wanted to touch me at the hospital, nobody wanted to explain how I lost my baby, perhaps they thought I was young and foolish," she recounted, her face staring into nothingness.

Tommy held her close, quiet, listening too to a tale he must have heard countless times, but which seemed fresh each time. Sad and painful. I sat still. Shaken.

"I have had seven pregnancies, all of them stillbirths, save one, a daughter...," she continued. A tear fell from Tommy's eye, another from me. But Waridi's face remained tearless, though grave. Despite the sadness, I was anxious to hear about the one that survived. I wanted to see her.

"But she died too, just when she turned sixteen," Waridi added, and for the first time, her eyes could not hold back the tears.

I was crushed. I wanted to run away. I had thought myself strong, but I could not handle this. It shook me to the core. How could one experience so much loss? I was angry at God; I was angry at myself. I was angry at Uncle Keroga.

"If it wasn't for Tommy, I would not be here, if only I could give him a child, just one who can grow and not die ...," she cried again and Tommy held her more closely.

Waridi turned to Tommy and thanked him, tears still falling from her eyes.

"After my surgery, the catheter I was given injured my urethra, I had allergies too. I lost hope again, I could not heal, I wanted out," Waridi continued. I was confused again; I did not understand what a catheter was and why it injured her.

Tommy must have sensed this and relieved his wife of the burden of an explanation. He illustrated this in the best way that he could.

It was difficult facing Waridi, her composure disturbed me, her concealed pain broke me. Despite her recovery, she was angry at how difficult it was to give birth to dead children while watching other women in the same room enjoy the joy of their newborns.

"It tortured me. I wished hospitals could have had different rooms for those who had lost their children..." she said bitterly. "The grieving need privacy, they need proper counselling, I was denied that..." Her anger was rising. But she was quick to check it before it could overwhelm her. With a smile, she turned to me and said, "But I am healed now, that is all that matters."

They stood, shook my hand again, with so much joy, and left for their periodic doctor's checkup.

I was broken.

Under the Heel of Fistula

At twenty-five years old, I am not a little girl anymore. Life has carved a fighter out of me. I am not the innocent soul that can easily fall for little gimmicks nor talk, no, not anymore. At twenty-five, I can be a mother, but I have chosen not to be one. I also know that with my position as a woman, the party and path to motherhood can easily come down to me. But motherhood is nothing new. At twelve, I was a mother to my mother and siblings. That was what life conspired to lay on my tiny hands. But again, that is life.

I vividly recall the Saturday afternoon when my uncle's Peugeot 404 pick-up truck drove into the compound. My three uncles, an aunt and two other neighbours were perched on the back, seated on the edge of the carrier.

As the vehicle parked, everyone scrambled off, as the passenger jerked the door back and forth. Suddenly, the passenger succeeded and finally opened the door. It was my mother. She looked jarred, her head drowning in a shawl. We stood there, dusty and befuddled. My little brother stared at me, as Mother passed us without saying a word. That was eerie.

Mum had left three days previously for the hospital, to deliver our brother. I might have been twelve years old or thereabouts, but I knew that Mum was expectant. I had watched as her belly grew from a mere bump to a huge bulge. She had also slowed down in a lot in her chores. Most of the work was handled by me and my brothers then aged ten and seven years.

We lived in Kapsaos near the famous Kapsaos market in Ainamoi division, Kericho District. Our home had a typical Kalenjin setting – a mud-walled main house and several grass-thatched huts. We also had plenty of livestock that were often taken care of by my younger brothers. Our village was adjacent to the famous tea estates run by Unilever. Previously, the holding company was called Brooke Bond. I still do not know when and why it changed names, not that it mattered to me anyway.

All I knew was that the tea estates had so many people from various parts of Kenya, who used to visit our market every first Monday of the month. Most would have received their monthly pay, and would prefer buying from our open-air market, which was considered cheap. They still do. Most of these buyers were tea pickers in the neighbouring Chagaik, Cheymen, Kipketer, Kimugu and Cheboswa Tea Estates. We all knew that they lived in squalor, in deplorable houses provided by the holding company.

My uncle, a shrewd businessman, used to trade with them. He used his pick-up to transport goods from Kericho Town to the market. He also ran a wholesale shop in the town. However, four of his brothers were dedicated drunkards. They included my father.

I call him a father, because he is my father. I dare call him a sperm donor. Looking back, I think this man, Joash Kiboi, only loved my mum when she had nothing on. He did not provide for us and would often turn the house into a World War Three theatre. We would suffer his beatings with Mum enduring it all. The Peugeot owner, my Uncle Tirop, would run to our house to calm the situation.… He had a way with his brother. Father would hurl abuses at him, but he would end the conflict. My father used to disappear from home into the tea estates for long and return smelling like a garbage truck, slump on the torn old seats in our house and snooze for hours. The snores could rattle a dead man to life. The booze-reeking breath would fill the house. Upon waking up, he would roughly demand to be given food. I still do not understand why Mum continued living with such a loafer who only served as a bad example for the younger generation.

In his absence, my uncle provided us with nearly everything that we needed. From basic home supplies to our books and pens and pencils, we all ran to him. He would always remind us to work hard in school.

During Mum's pregnancy, he took her to the hospital once. When they returned, Mum excitedly told us that she was carrying a baby boy. Another brother for us. I was the only girl.

However, Mum was a feeder. Our grandmother and aunts would bring her loads and loads of food. From milk, eggs, to porridge, Mum would be encouraged to eat to be strong. And this, she successfully did. Initially, she was slender and tall. But by the time she was heading to the hospital with Uncle Tirop, she was as chubby as a pig. One would have confused her with a small hut.

So here we were, dusty village kids, some with runny noses, waiting for the news.

As the last man alighted, he joined the rest in receiving a box. That was when I realized that something was amiss. I ran to my uncle and asked him where the baby was… He silently pointed to the box. I froze.

"Chela," Aunty Rosa called me. Chela is my pet name. It is the short form of Chelagat, my full name. "Please come." Her voice was authoritative. Aunty Rosa was married to Uncle Tirop.

As I peeled myself from my siblings to join Aunty, she met me midway and held my hand. She then led me behind the granary and stopped before bending over my small frame. "Mama has lost the baby … your brother. She was in too much pain and they had to pull the boy out. He was very big. Four kilogrammes. We have come to bury the body here," she said.

That was the moment tears welled in my eyes. I let them flow. I sat on one of the stones that supported the granary and cried for as long as I could recall. I just sat there, dazed and confused. I imagined how my brother would have turned out. Tall? Athletic? Chocolate-skinned like me or a brownie like Mum? I could not stop thinking about whom he would look like. I also imagined the heavenly world – the after world. Was it always sunny, golden sunny or just dark? How cruel was it that one could just die before seeing the world down here? Well, death had its own equalizing power. But what was it balancing when it ripped such a young life from this world? As I sat lost in my thoughts, Aunty Rosa returned and grabbed my hand.

"Come on, Chela, you need to change. The priest has arrived and we need to finish the ceremony soon. Your mum needs to return to hospital, for cleaning," she said as I walked behind her.

The service was short and curt. There were more prayers than songs. No eulogy for the dead baby. No colourful words to describe his nature, for he had no known temperament. Not even the flow of tears except from my mother and myself. Just a small gathering from a local African Inland Church. My Kalenjin community was not known to be overly dramatic over death. Wails did not alert a passer-by to the home of the bereaved. The loss of a loved one was usually expressed through muted sobs and equally hushed lamentations about the gap left by the departed.

On this day, Mum's sobs were louder than usual for she was the only adult grieving. What could the rest be mourning? The little boy was a soldier of fate, who died in a vicious battle he neither knew nor remembered. All that mattered was that he fought, lost, rested and was now playing in heavenly bliss, peace and happiness. Amid seraph joy, he rested.

My little brother's corpse was in a Kenya Cooperative Creameries milk carton, which was fully covered with the upper flaps slid into each other with no string to hold them up. The body could have been removed from the freezers, as the carton showed signs of moisture, a sign of a thawing in the searing sun. The bundle sat desolately on a rickety table, capturing the sombre mood that engulfed the moment. Rural misery that rides on soaking poverty.

Just as the priest was finishing the final prayer before proceeding to the grave, everyone was rattled by a thunderous voice. "Who else... I ask... Who else...? Who else is married to a white woman apart from myself Joash Kiboi?!" That was my dad. A seasoned civil servant who served his water ministry with dedication for a whopping 30 years.

Despite the situation, everyone burst into laughter. Uncle Tirop and two of our distant uncles rushed towards the entrance. My father was home. He had disappeared for days on his drinking sojourns in the estates.

He must have been unaware of the calamity that had befallen his family for a few minutes later, he was dragged to the graveside, afflicted and drenched in sorrow and tears.

Later, the priest finished the final rites and we all headed to the main house for a meal. Father was taken straight to bed.

"He was a little giant," Mama said sombrely. "I endured painful labour for three hours at the clinic. A nurse, assisted by your uncle, finally decided to pull out the baby. He was dead. But he tipped 4 kilogrammes on the scales. The doctor blamed it on my diet during my pregnancy. I used to eat like a pig!"

She also added that the body of my brother was placed on a little table beside her bed for thirty minutes, for her to have her closure. "He resembled your father. Your uncle is the one who placed the body on the table." My heart was battered.

My dad slept for twelve straight hours until the following day. Then he woke up, barked at everyone and headed out... maybe to forget his sorrow with a cold Tusker.

Mother walked to my uncle's Peugeot and headed to the clinic, for what they referred to as 'cleaning'. That was when I noticed that she was limping, and her clothes were drenched...

Uncle Tirop brought Mum back the following day. I do not know what happened at the clinic, but the woman who was carried from the vehicle was clearly not my mother. I still feel like Mum was left behind and a badly-crippled female version of her delivered to us.

Mum was paralysed on her left leg. She could not walk on her own. From that day onwards, Mum became my baby. We literally switched roles. I assumed the responsibility of taking care of her. She could neither move nor sit. Her lower limbs were numb, cold and pale. She was also always passing urine and faecal matter. Imagine cleaning your mother's poop ... the stench, the murky sight ... and the psychological mess.

With my father's erratic behaviour and disappearing acts, Uncle Tirop was left with the responsibility of providing us with daily incidentals. I was the mother of the house. I had to seek permission from my school to be arriving late and even leaving class sessions to attend to Mum. My teachers were very understanding. The headteacher, Mr Songok, would sometimes accompany me to help me move my mother around.

I recall how one day it rained heavily. I had taken my mum to bask outside. Still a little child, I completely forgot about her. I found Mother choking on rainwater, as she wallowed in the mire of rainwater mixed with urine and poop. I am sure that she swallowed part of her waste. Her bedding was caked in mud and faecal matter. She caught one of her worst colds in the aftermath of that mess. I lit a huge fire and spread her near it. The wet firewood produced so much smoke that one could easily have confused it with Hell's fire. Mother coughed through it. But she was warm.

I have never forgiven myself. No one at home cared to check on her. From that day onwards, teachers would often remind me to check on her. I even grew muscles from dragging Mum around. However, she was very grateful to me and uses that incident to hail my caring side.

One day, a friend of Mum's passed by with some herbs. I still do not know how they worked or whether to believe that they worked. But a few days after rubbing and massaging the concoction on her legs and lower back, sensitivity started returning to her lower limbs. In a few days, Mum was walking a bit slowly with a walking stick. However, her involuntary flow of faecal matter and urine had not stopped. Within this period, I watched as my mother shrunk from a mother, to a cripple with a crushed self-esteem. Even after regaining some walking ability, her ego was completely crushed. The evil talk and bad-mouthing from people had played a big role in hampering her complete recovery. I was overly happy for her for the progress. She was not.

A few days after my twenty-fourth birthday, a female supervisor from the Cheymen Tea Plantation visited to check on Mum's last goat that she had intended to buy. The mountains of fabric that Mum had placed between her legs got soaked and dropped to the ground, creating splotches in the sand. As adults around us fanned their noses while walking away, I picked the dirty secret and ran towards the house. I had the responsibility of covering my mother's personal shame. My mother stood still, mortified. Meanwhile, more murk flowed down her legs into the sand.

When I returned, I found them talking.

"Don't worry. I think you have a hole in you. My daughter is a nurse. I hear them calling this condition fistula," she was saying.

From her accent, she was from Western Kenya. We studied with children from that region from the estates. So, I knew this. She continued, "There is an upcoming clinic at the Kericho District Hospital for women with this condition. Please go there and find out when it will take place."

When Uncle Tirop arrived, we did not let him rest. We shared the news and he agreed follow it up the next morning. We were shocked when he arrived back the following day at around 10 a.m. He was panting. He gave Mum ten minutes to prepare. Registration and screening of patients was happening on the same day and we had no time to waste.

On the way, he drove like a mad man. Some wily police officers stopped us. One of them boarded our vehicle, squeezing Mum and myself in the process. He then ordered him to drive to a nearby police station. Some Kenyan police officers have been topping all statistics as far as taking of bribes is concerned. Uncle, completely irritated by the officer's failure to listen to him, drove the vehicle straight to the county's police headquarters, and called the commander. It turned out that they were friends. When the male officer saw his senior, he bolted out like an antelope. We were left laughing. Interestingly, Mum had stained his clothes!

After pleasantries with the commander, he reversed the car and headed straight to the hospital. We were the second last to be attended to. Mum was registered and screened. She was told to report back after two weeks for admission. Those were the longest two weeks we have ever endured.

When Mum was wheeled into the theatre, I prayed to God to save her. I told Him to work through the doctors from Nairobi, to manifest Himself to mankind and to those who spat at Mum. And to allow me a testimony as I looked forward to a new world. At twenty-four years old, I had attended day primary and secondary schools around the village. My strained studies never saw me muster a good score. But I did not regret it. I was determined to achieve something big. Temporary abandonment from my dad had degenerated into insults and spite. Epithets had brought forth slaps and beatings.

"An adult woman who wets herself," he would growl. Mother's screams would be her defence, for Uncle Tirop would arrive and calm the situation. Dad always slept on his rickety couches whenever Uncle was around.

Two weeks after the surgery, Mum was discharged. I had used the little money I had earned from doing laundry for some well-off neighbours to buy her new bedding. We had joined hands with my siblings in cleaning up our house, scrubbing every nook and cranny of her bedroom. The room transformed and became sparkling clean. When Mum walked into the house, our eyes were fixed to her ankles. Hallelujah! Nothing was flowing. No whiff of odour. My mother was clean! She still is.

One year later, I moved from home to Eldoret, where I work for a transport company in the logistics department. I have managed to renovate our house. Dad is now reformed and both have joined the church. It is a new beginning. But I am sorry to state that I am too damaged to be any man's wife. However, I look back at my journey with Mum and my siblings, and clearly understand the lyrics of the good old country song, 'In The Good Old Days When Times Were Bad'. Like our Mount Kenya brothers and sisters, my Kalenjin people do love country music. I do.

Fistula and the Permanent Marital Fissure

I thought my marriage was made in heaven. I still thought it was, until I flunked it. Look, as a man, there comes a point in life when you become true to yourself, by loving thyself, appreciating your strengths, conquests and above all, the foolish mistakes that ride on your often-denied weaknesses.

As a carpenter, I learnt to live and work to perfection. It is one acquired trait that one must live by to survive in this trade. Nothing should go wrong, and getting something perfect should be any craftsman's sole dedication. After all, this is one profession appreciated in the holy writ.

My name is John Njeru. Some call me Njesh, for my fame around Siakago, in Embu, is two-fold. I am famous for being the local man who perfected a trade inspired by Jesus' father, carpentry. I once ran a successful workshop whose works adorn both poor and Grecian homes and business premises of countless locals. But that was when it thrived. Now, it thrives on a colourful memory, as it slumbers in its rot. Apart from that, I also live in infamy for being a marital nincompoop.

My tribulations started when my beautiful wife, Winnie, was five months pregnant with our second baby. Ours was a marriage conjured up in heaven, confirmed in hell as true and played out in this world, in my house.

Winnie was the jewel that any man would have died for to have as a wife. With Somali hair, an Embu face, Maasai teeth and a Luo figure, what else would a man want in life? It took me days and eons of cajoling to make her fall for me. And in marriage, she was a perfect mother, with a golden brain and an equally golden heart full of love, and a laid-back disposition that harboured nothing but blissful care for our daughter and myself. She was my queen.

She quit her job as a nursery school teacher in a local private school to run the poultry business that I had set up for her. This followed my flourishing carpentry business that saw me expand my workshop within Siakago Town.

While both of us are from Embu, I hail from Siakago, while she is from Kiang'ombe, in Embu North. We both are from the Mbeere community, which is part of the larger Embu County.

Well, in the fifth month of her pregnancy, we started noticing her bleeding. Sometimes, the bleeding would be heavy, accompanied by huge blood clots. That was scary! We went to a local clinic, where doctors said that there was nothing to worry about. However, she was warned against taking on strenuous chores. As the days dragged on, she started complaining that the baby was more docile than our first born. I assured her that these children were two different individuals with independent personalities, and we she should have avoided the temptation of comparing them, even after the baby's arrival.

The scans had indicated that she was carrying a boy, which sent a thrill down my knees, since, as an African man, I planned to name him after my late dad. Although times had changed, my community still put a lot of importance on sons. It was a twisted ideology, yet so African. Sons inherit their fathers. And in the case of the death of the man of the house, a son assumes the role of his father, based on the saying that 'a son is as good as his father'.

I recall vividly when her labour pains kicked in. She was eight months into the pregnancy. It caught both of us by surprise one evening at around 9 p.m. I rushed her to the local clinic. As she was wheeled into the delivery room, the feisty nurses barked at me to let them do their job. I was left with no option but to head home. I returned the following morning only to find my Winnie still in pain, wailing and cursing me for putting her in the family way. Any man who has been in such a situation knows how sweet those insults can be. African women do have choice expletives for husbands whenever they are in labour. Interestingly, the irony is that they soon forget the pain after the arrival of their bundles of joy!

Epithets aside, Winnie was also badly exhausted. This depressed me.

On the fifth day, I was almost bursting with rage when nurses told me that her birth canal was yet to open. Five days!

After I ranted like Lucifer's first disciple, they wheeled her into the theatre. An hour later, my son was delivered through Caesarean section, but immediately put into the nursery. My wife was too weak to even speak, she had endured a lot of pain during the prolonged labour and being light-skinned, she had turned pink.

For close to six days, I would wake up to go check on my family. I would first pass by the workshop, inspect the progress of tasks, assign new ones and proceed to the hospital. I would always find my wife asleep, check on the baby, then stay by Winnie's bedside until she woke up. Her first words were always about the baby. I would assure her that the baby was in the nursery. But she was not always convinced.

On the last day, I was shocked to find our son missing from the nursery. A rotund nurse rudely told me that the baby had passed away that morning, then wobbled away.

I was shocked, bitter and drained. I had big plans for the boy. I had even chosen his name – Peter Ndwiga. That is my late father's name. I wailed like a baby. My wife saw me crying and immediately enquired about the baby. I just told her plainly that the baby was dead. Another nurse confirmed the news to her. She howled, yowled and keened in grief. Her breasts out, hands in air and her feet stamping like an agitated bull, hers was the bitter cry of a mother.

I later stepped out of the clinic and called my brother, who informed the rest of the family. In less than an hour, they arrived with a simple carton that was lined with a folded piece of blanket. My son's stiff little body was wrapped in a simple white cloth. It had a creamish stain of mucus on the lower edge – a last indicator of my little son's desperate struggle to stay alive. My mother received the body, turned to me and placed it in my arms. It felt cold and light. Everyone else then stepped back. My hands started trembling. Anger started building in me, then sorrow engulfed me. My heart was hollow, an emptiness that I am yet to fill.

"Here. Speak your last words to your son. He was from your loins," Mother said tearfully.

That was bizarre. I held the boy and unwrapped his face. It had black spots. His chest was also slightly visible. I realized my loss. His hands were stretched down along his body. Stiff.

"Son, the moment we shared was brief. Thank you for allowing us to be your parents during your short, but troubled journey in this world. Go well, and intervene for us," I whispered as I made the sign of the cross because I am Catholic. Later, Mum appeared with teary eyes and grabbed the body from me. She placed it in the box and covered it with a shawl. My brother lifted it and walked a short distance to my uncle's Toyota Probox. I walked right behind him. The boot was opened and the carton placed inside. I was escorted by my mother and sat on the back left seat of the same car. On the short drive home, I kept stealing glances at the carton, as thoughts of my wife flooded my mind.

At home, a local Catholic priest joined us and led a short funeral mass for our departed son. I had to give the hospital management the proposed name of the infant, which was later entered into the stillbirth certificate. Everything was happening so fast and felt eerie. In less than an hour, we were done. No one else attended the gloomy ceremony apart from the immediate family. I headed back to the hospital to see Winnie. I found her breathing heavily in deep slumber. She had been sedated.

I visited Winnie every day. She had been admitted over an undisclosed complication, allegedly occasioned by the prolonged labour. None of the hospital staff was willing to reveal the issue to us. However, I noticed that whenever I met Winnie, she walked with a funny gait. It seemed like she was trudging while hauling a heavy load between her legs. There was also some discomfort about her. She was ashamed of seeing me. My complaints fell on deaf ears.

One morning, I walked in unannounced. I was shocked to see my wife standing, with urine welling around the soles of her slippers. I just could not comprehend what was happening. I confronted the nurses on duty. One of them told me that my wife had raptured her bladder due to the prolonged labour.

"And why didn't you inform me earlier?" I thundered.

They all went mute. They must have sensed danger, because they silently left, one followed by another. Kenyan hospitals are manned by well-trained staff but some are way too heartless to care.

The following day, I transferred her to the Embu Level Four Hospital, where she was operated on after two days, and stayed for three weeks. The surgery left one of her legs numb. Jeez! This now caused me more and more psychological strain. My Winnie could not walk! She could only move around in a wheelchair. My Winnie…

Wheelchair aside, the urine did not stop flowing. On being discharged, we were warned against sex for three months to allow her to heal well.

At home, my darling Winnie was a mess. The smell of urine was unbearable. She had to literally stash mountains and mountains of linen on her side of the bed, to avoid saturating the mattress with pee. Every morning, she would embark on washing the cloths for the next night. Whenever they failed to dry, she opted to use them while still wet. I was forced to buy her more materials for switching. The acrid smell in the room was too much to take. Friends and relatives who used to flock into our house every day, stopped. They were all nauseated by the odour. I watched as Winnie's self-esteem took a hit. I always tried to encourage her but she was too preoccupied with her troubles. She was inconsolable.

I would cry when alone. She stopped attending church. She was always withdrawn, with nasty mood swings that resulted in bitter altercations between us. She would refuse my offers to help where possible, and would bark at me to let her be. She thought that I was ridiculing her. My relatives stayed away, as she was too hostile towards them. I decided to offer the little emotional and physical help I could to my wife, while trying as much as possible to give her space. This was really frustrating. This bellicose Winnie was a stranger to me.

During one of her many clinic visits to Embu Level Four Hospital, a certain medic referred us to a Dr Munyoki who is based at the St. Mary's Hospital in Langata. We arrived at the hospital three days later. He performed the surgery, which saw Winnie spend another three weeks in the ward, but to no success. Again, we were asked to avoid sex for three months. That made it half a year for myself. Pressure!

Back home, things were not working well. I turned to the bottle. To escape my trouble, I embraced imbibing and what came with it. Soon, a nubile girl happened between us. I started pestering Winnie to allow me to have another woman that I could have sex with to relieve the pressure in me. Shockingly, Winnie obliged. She even offered to move to another bedroom, and allow me and my new catch to use our bedroom. I bought a new bed and bedding and settled in. However, I never allowed the women to hang around the house when I was away.

They were paid prostitutes who were there to serve their short-term purpose. Winnie was stone-faced. She never even spoke to the women. Never blamed me. She was just in her own world, dazed and mutely confused. Like a drenched person to whom cold water does not cause discomfort, she was emotionally numb. I could always see her pain but I guess I was too wrecked to care.

It had been three years since our marital challenges began. Three years since my marriage assumed a twisted position. My first-born daughter was living with one of my wife's sisters. She had been taken away to allow us to deal with the frequent hospital trips. I also believed that Winnie had informed her family of the odd marital alignments in her house, thus they opted to keep the girl away from this very unpleasant place that was our house.

It was in this third year, that yet another proposal came through Dr Munyoki, who had operated on my wife at St. Mary's Hospital. He proposed that we try a fistula camp at the Kenyatta National Hospital. We did. Too bad! We never managed to meet any specialist there. The red tape there could easily beat the Chinese politburo bureaucracy! We gave up and went back to our usual marital spectacle. By then, my finances were messed up. My workshop was almost collapsing as clients reduced and my carpenters decided to steal from me. I could not afford to pay them, since the money had gone into Winnie's medical bills, alcohol and prostitutes. They had their reasons to steal from me, to pay themselves. I struggled with bills. Even purchasing diapers for my wife became a challenge. She would use one diaper after every twenty minutes. Each diaper cost Ksh 150 ($1.50).

Three months after the last failed surgery, I came back home with my lass, only to find my wife missing. I chased away the new woman, as I desperately tried to find Winnie. I searched for her in every corner of the house. I called all her friends that I knew. None of them had any idea of her whereabouts. All her clothes were missing, just like her personal effects were. I could not call her sisters because they had developed a nasty attitude towards me. To them, I was to blame for their sister's predicament. They maintained that I was not doing enough for their sibling. They saw me as a failed husband, and they were right.

The women I had brought to my house for the nightly romps had picked our dirty little secret and broadcasted it to my drinking buddies. I was the centre of their nasty jokes. To them, I was this failure with a worthless wife. A woman who pees in bed like a child! I was this character called 'Kabogogi' whose failures are hilariously enumerated in a song by Kikuyu Benga star, Kariuki wa Kiarutara. I was the cursed one who soaked in my wife's urine every evening. Some even claimed that I wore my wife's panties like a woman and carried babies on my back in shawls like a girl. I was the Njeru who could not mount his wife. He who had ceded his marital bed to prostitutes of Embu… Hell!

The stigma busted my ego. I would get into fights in clubs. I had very many assault cases at the local police station, which translated to more payments to settle the cases out of court. Police officers did not hear my side of story, because, according to Kenyan law, in cases of assault, whoever was reported first was the offender. Blast the law! I would in turn vent my anger on Winnie. It was not once nor twice that I assaulted her. I would slap her just to convince myself that I was the man of the house. She never answered me. She would stare at me, silently, as tears rolled down her cheeks.

As these memories flowed back, a nasty sense of guilt descended into my heart. I cried for hours as I recalled the vows I had made in church on our wedding day. How I had promised to love, to cherish and to hold; for better for worse, for richer for poorer, in sickness and in health …. In sickness and in health …. The last words kept ringing in my head as reality checked in. I was a flawed piece of God's art. A conflicted spirit with no sense of moral direction, which could not fit into a social order. A failed father. A failed husband. A failed friend. A failed businessman. A failure in stilts. I had let my Winnie down. The vows I made before God, all broken by a fistula. The hole in Winnie that created the mess had grown into a rift that had consumed my marriage, because I had allowed it. I let my Winnie down at a time she needed me most: in her sickness. I assaulted my sick wife. God!

I do not know how and when I passed out. But I was woken up by a stray dog, licking my face. It was cleaning the vomit around my mouth. A dog's life….

Winnie disappeared for almost three weeks. I later learnt that she had been admitted to a facility called Family Health, where she had undergone a successful surgery. Her brother had facilitated her trip to Nairobi. I wondered why they never looped me in, but understood her desperation. I could not blame her, hence hoped that she would return. I could not wait to receive her back home. A visiting Malawian doctor performed the operation.

I stopped bringing women home and cleaned the house thoroughly. I replaced her bedding and all her clothes. The house was now fresh and sparkling clean. I later travelled to Nairobi, in search of the facility. It was like searching for a needle in a haystack. Three days later, I walked into the hospital. Upon enquiry, I was informed that she had been discharged. I immediately headed back home, only to be welcomed by a clean but empty house.

Winnie never returned. It has been three years now since the new era. I have not seen my daughter since then. I only bumped into one of my wife's sisters, who sneered and spit in contempt. I understood Winnie and her siblings' anger. Fistula had created a fissure in my marriage that later grew into a fault that swallowed our bond. Looking back, I realize how ignorance can consume our best. Look, I am an educated man. I just failed to seek proper advice. Had I taken the initiative, I would not have fallen by the wayside. I would have been there for my Winnie. I had done so well, but slacked midway. I should not have trusted that clinic…

I have since read a lot about fistula and realized that it is a common condition caused by our failures as a society. Our governance issues have played into the existing chaotic approach to fistula. I have since been involved in sensitizing the community on fistula, its causes and available treatment options. As I write this, I have joined hands with fellow local businessmen to facilitate a fistula camp at the Embu County Hospital. I may never have my Winnie back, but my efforts will save another marriage somewhere, anywhere. Well, my workshop is rising from the ashes.

Joy's Rise from the Ashes

After leaving the Bustani Rehabilitation Centre in Nairobi, I decided to pick up the remaining pieces of my life by taking up a teaching job in a private school situated in western Kenya. Mine was a life of bad choices with deserved consequences. I had lost my home to auctioneers, abandoned my job and was in turn abandoned by my wife and two lovely children. My second born has Caucasian features. I still feel that I was too wasted to sire. So, my wife could have out-sourced the seed. She becomes defensive whenever I question the source of these genes. All in all, I had also turned into a hopeless junky who depended on his wife and commanded no respect from my own children. They could not take it any more.

To steer clear of drugs, alcohol and women, I had no choice but to stay away from bad company. Out of my six friends, four were dead and the remaining two were graves-in-waiting. I was lucky to have been the survivor. But that is life, as we would say every time we buried one of us.

Landing in Bungoma was easy and I effortlessly met and started making new friends. One such friend was a radiant lady called Joy. Joy ran a grocery shop at the Chepkube open-air market. She caught my attention through her dressing. She dressed in what could unsettle my liberal Kiambu society, whose daughters were thought to be overboard. During our conversations as she chopped my traditional vegetables, she would barely speak two sentences without exalting her husband. This would leave a void in my heart, as I recalled how my wife had walked away due to my disastrous ways. She left with our children, house girl and all our belongings. I could never imagine her waxing lyrical about me. Yet, here was a woman, wallowing in poverty but still proud of her husband.

Whenever I asked her why her husband made her tick, she would excitedly say, *"Wa moja havai mbili. Wangu ni wangu."* Loosely translated, it meant, 'He who wears one pair of clothes, cannot wear two. My husband is my husband." I was taken in by her mastery of the Swahili language. As far as was concerned, my Central Kenya folks had a troubled relationship with this wonderful African language.

Bungoma is one of the frontier western Kenya counties. It is also the corridor to countries within the Great Lakes Region. It is dominated by the Luhya community, with the Bukusu sub-tribe making up the majority of the native population. Bungoma also has a good number of investors from other parts of Kenya, especially from Kakamega and Central Kenya, Somalis and even those of Asian descent. It is also an agricultural hub responsible for maize production, apart from being part of the Western Kenya sugar belt. The local Bukusu are related to Uganda's Bagisu people, with whom they share a lot of traditions. The Bukusus are also known to be traditional, whose lives are guided by a strict adherence to customs and rites, unlike the other Luhya sub-tribes. Their circumcision ceremonies are not only colourful but also famous.

This is the ethnic group that Joy belongs to. On this day, she had promised to share her story. And to create more time, she brought along a hand to take care of her business. "My husband is wonderful, because he foolishly married and stuck to a stinking woman. I really don't think he had experience with those pretty urban women who don't emit a whiff. I might have been this lucky to meet what you Nairobi men could easily refer to as 'inexperienced'. I believe he thought that was how women should smell."

"What?" I interjected.

"Listen, I want to believe that you came here to listen to me talk about my life…"

"Yes, yes," I said as I bowed shamefully. In my earlier days, I could have snapped. But I was a changed man now.

"Then why are you interrupting me?"

That was a subtle order for me to shut my mouth. I nodded in embarrassment and clasped my hands, a sign of submission. Here is her story in her words:

"See, I fell pregnant while staying with my cousin in Langata in Nairobi. Despite being in primary school, I did flirt with a man and the soil splattered on me. I could not tell my cousin about it. A month into my pregnancy, I asked her to let me go back home to Bungoma. She was puzzled, since I had not told her about the life growing inside me.

"Upon arriving here, I went straight to my maternal grandmother's place in Chwele, since my mother was not around. There, I found that my granny had also relocated to her other home in Shivembe. I stayed for a few days, under the care of my maternal uncle.

"My uncle is a calamitous character who has sunk deep into alcoholism. His life is a waste. He used to vent his frustrations on me by physically abusing and threatening to rape me, together with one of my female cousins.

"Sometimes, we were forced to spend the nights in sugarcane and sorghum plantations as the constant harassment grew each day. I later escaped to his daughter's place and disclosed my being in the family way. She warned me against incurring an abortion. But deep down, I was determined to get rid of the pregnancy. I bought washing detergent and a packet of tea leaves. My cousin's sixth sense must have alerted her of my plans. She again persuaded me to abandon my plans. I complied.

"I later began attending antenatal clinics at the Chwele District Hospital. During one of my visits, the medics informed me that I was carrying a big child and that I should go for an elective Caesarean section delivery. They even gave me the dates.

"I grew more scared as the dates approached. I even started missing the days of my mistreatment in the hands of my uncle, since I felt that I deserved it. I stayed until my water broke and labour pains followed. I then headed for the hospital.

"I literally crawled into the facility, having sprained my ankle along the way. I was rushed into the operation theatre without processing. Mine was an emergency. Doctors and support staff worked very hard. But fate had its ugly way. As the doctor and nurses struggled, a power blackout hit the hospital. Despite the challenge, the medics finally managed to retrieve the foetus. The baby was immediately put on an oxygen machine, but I was immediately informed that it had died. Baby weighed a whopping 5.3 kilogrammes! Due to exhaustion, the baby had even passed stool while still in the womb.

"As information filtered to the village that I had lost my baby, family members trickled in. One by one, they passed by my bed, mumbling their condolences. I was too weak to attend the short funeral. I understand that my younger brother, who was then in high school, carried the corpse of his young nephew by hand. The family later buried the baby in a carton, in a grave that was later flattened. My mother, who had reappeared from God-knows-where, later returned to my ward and broke the bad news: that I would never have children, now that I had had a stillbirth. She tenuously blamed me for the death of my boy child. Mum was the last relative to visit me.

"I stayed in hospital for two months. For days, I relied on leftovers from my fellow patients. I had to depend on well-wishers for survival. But that was not the issue. What unsettled me was the endless involuntary flow of urine and faecal matter down my thighs, ankles and onto the floor. My bed was always soiled. The stench that I emitted could resurrect a corpse! My bills were piling. The more I stayed, the more I realized that I would never know peace, even in death. I was sure that the hospital would have detained my body had I attempted to die in their wards.

"Amidst the loss and desperation, God provided angels through some of the hospital staff. One nurse would always bring me hot meals whenever she was on duty. She also organized for some of her colleagues to donate to me some of their clothes and towels. Due to my leaking, I really needed such to try and maintain my hygiene.

"One particular morning, as the doctors were doing their rounds, the one who had attended to me the day I was admitted to the hospital was in the team. When they reached my bed, the lead doctor turned to him and said, "Dr Barasa, you see how you messed up this child? That was very wrong of you." They then walked away. Dr Barasa said nothing apart from glancing at me. That is the moment I realized that whatever could go wrong, had indeed gone wrong with me. See? Apart from my leaking urine and faecal matter, I also had a hole whose origin I still could not comprehend. It oozed blood, pus and other flesh-like substances that smelt like a thousand dead rats!

"One day, a white man appeared at the hospital. He must have either been a missionary or a charity worker. Upon speaking to some patients, he offered to offset their medical bills. I was one of them. He paid my Ksh 27,000 ($ 270) bill. He later tried to convince me to accompany him to Europe. I rejected the proposal. I was too careful with men after my experience with the man in Nairobi. They say once bitten, twice shy.

"When I was discharged, I took my stinky self back home. I was distraught, imagining that my son was buried somewhere in our compound. I later requested to be shown to his grave. Lo! When my brother took me to the site, we were all shocked to find that the body had been exhumed by stray dogs. Only a skull remained of the boy I neither saw nor held in my arms. It had been gnawed to pink! That hurt me deeply. Later on, as memories flashed through my mind, my breasts started oozing milk. My brother later reburied the only evidence of my son's short stint in this troubled world.

"Life outside the four walls of the hospital ward was nothing but a keg of rejection, dejection and humiliation. Everyone who saw me spat in disgust. None hesitated to remind me that I was reeking. Urine mixed with stool would stream endlessly. It took less than two minutes after any meal for the repulsive fluids to discharge. I would bathe up to four times each day. Nothing changed. Sometimes, the liquid would assume the smell of the food I ate. I used layers and layers of cloth to absorb the murk.

"I also tried as much as possible to stay away from public spaces. Some locals accused me of being a witch. I avoided attending funerals. However, I was dedicated to the church, although I would stay for less than thirty minutes in each service. To have an easy time in church, I would avoid taking fluids for up to four days beforehand. This somehow reduced the flow of urine and faecal matter. Some villagers even claimed that I was suffering from HIV and AIDS, which still led to stigma in most rural areas in Kenya. My skin would sometimes shed due to the loss of body fluids. This would leave me weak and unable to perform heavy chores. I was forced to move from one place to another to avoid humiliation. I recall how I was forced to flee my grandmother's place, after she organized to marry me off to a man as old as a god.

"One day, I bumped into a man – my current husband. He seemed really interested in me. No matter how hard I tried to avoid him, he kept reaching out to me. We dated for almost one year, and later got married. Throughout our dating period, I tried as much as I could to keep my 'dirty issues' away from him.

"Our sex life was a painful experience for me. I would create a mountain of cloth to avoid soiling the bed. Whenever we made love, he would be left wondering why I emitted so much fluid from my reproductive organs. I could also tell that he had thoughts about my smell, but he kept it all to himself.

"With him, we have three children. One day, our firstborn daughter came back from school and openly asked me why I do not observe hygiene. This hurt me deeply. It was her first cut into my emotional flesh, and it ran deep. Whenever the smell was too much for her, I would pretend to have broken wind, then cunningly blame it on her. The girl was also bullied in school over my condition.

"Amid prayer and hope, I played hide and seek with my husband until the second and third children were born. I would sometimes make short visits to some of our friends' homes and leave after completely using their toilet rolls to cover my flows.

"One day, I visited my sister-in-law. I had heard about a fistula clinic at the Kenyatta National Hospital on Radio Citizen. I asked her for help, which she did. She gave me money for transport and other needs.

"The following day, armed with my rags, towels and other linen, I boarded a bus headed to Bungoma Town, and later connected to Nairobi.

"Upon reaching Kenyatta National Hospital, I was processed and given an invoice for payment. But I was startled when, upon presenting the invoice to a senior doctor, he tore it up and ushered me in. What shocked me was the sheer number of women from different parts of Kenya who had similar, if not worse, conditions. We were informed that we had fistula. Doctors Khisa and Sabina took each patient through the steps on how fistulas develop, what causes them and how the surgeries would help us.

"The following day, I was on the surgical table. As the anaesthesia took effect, all my past experiences came flowing back, like a nightmare, they appeared real. I really thought that I had overcome them, but, like the angel of death, they were still haunting me. Then darkness descended on me.

"I woke up the following morning in a hospital ward. This traumatized me, as I started screaming. A friendly nurse ran to my bedside and assured me that it was over. Dr Khisa later passed by and laughed reassuringly as I thanked him for allowing himself to be God's helping hand to suffering humanity.

"Two weeks later, we were discharged. What shocks me up to now, is the fact that I can wear any attire of my choice. I can walk around in dry clothes. I do not even wet my underwear. I wear all fashionable styles that I missed, just for my husband. I please no one, but him … for as I said, he loved me when I was avoided by all, when I was smelling like a discredited morgue. Now, I make myself look and smell good, just for him."

Joy's narration ended, as she did a little catwalk on the pavement.

The woman's story shocked me. I stared at her in bewilderment.

"How old were you when you fell pregnant?" I asked her.

"I was still in primary school, around thirteen years."

"And the man responsible?"

"He was a construction worker."

"Do you know where he is?"

"No. But am just happy. I care less about him now. That is in the past. My periods are now back, I can now enjoy sex and interact with people without fear and shame. My self-esteem is way up there," she said, pointing to the sky.

As I walked away to my abode, I could not help reflecting on the journey trod by Joy. Hers is a relief, having been there with fistula, lived it and braved through it. Now, she rides on hope and happiness. And with her new-found freedom, I can only seek inspiration from her, as I guide my students through the journey of life, and turn a new page. Remember, I was once a wreck. Now, under construction. Motherhood need not be condemnation. This is what I will teach my boys. They are the ones who will, in future, marry and live with women who may be victims of fistula. I will teach these boys to always stand with their women. To refrain from stigmatizing those affected by this condition. To research, and understand that fistula is treatable. It is not a curse. Neither is it witchcraft. Fistula rides on poverty, lack of information and poor governance.

$$Part\ 3$$

Stories narrated by medical caregivers

•◦• ● •◦•

Insights of Healthcare Workers

Background

In most African countries, healthcare providers are the primary source of health information. Because of the low doctor-population ratio in the continent, it is the other cadre of healthcare providers that interact with patients more often. For instance, majority of deliveries are conducted by midwives and nurses more often than doctors. The danger for these women often lies in the truth that most healthcare providers are not as informed as they should be when it comes to complex cases such as obstetric fistula. This is even as patients look up to them for information. However, because of the strong social position of children in the African culture, many healthcare providers work hard and do their best despite the challenges they face. The narratives in this chapter dig into obstetric fistula and stillbirth events from the standpoint of healthcare providers.

A Bird's-Eye View

I would watch their hearts break. I would hear their voiceless cries, the cries of the soul when there were no more tears to shed. Most just wanted to talk, to be listened to, to be reassured of love and understanding. To some, the hospital beds were their sanctuary at a time when society could not endure them with their leakages, thanks to fistula. But for some, the hospital was their nightmare. A constant reminder of where they lost their children, some of whose voices they never heard. The cries of the newborns that were the result of successful deliveries, with all outward signs that they would survive to see their children, disturbed those who had lost theirs. It was a tragedy that they had to be in the same room. It would break my heart to the extent that I could not talk or listen to those who wanted an ear, and solace. There was no privacy.

But I had a duty as nurse; to reassure them of their healing, to give hope to those that lost theirs in whichever way I could, even where circumstances did not favour then greatly. I hated it when I had to break the news to them, "The child did not make it, the child died."

"Nurse Mogire…," someone called me from the waiting area as I entered the reception to clock in at work.

It was a dark, shy-faced short lady. She smiled beautifully. But it was a smile that had seen and defied suffering for long. One that had seen pain in all its dull colours. The many years I had served as a nurse had taught me so much about pain and suffering. I could read it in a voice, in laughter and in people's walking styles. I could tell those who masked their pain behind a stern indifference to the world. I could read rejection behind a disturbing thirst for power and money.

"I am Maureen, you helped me during my first pregnancy," she said, her smile broadening further.

It had been nine years since the pregnancy in question. How time flies! She looked older than she really was.

"Oh, happy to see you. It has been long; how is your son?" I inquired.

She smiled then paused to take in some breath. She smiled again, but this time, her eyes welled up with tears which she rushed to conceal with her hands. I put my hand around her and escorted her to the office

I shared with Sister Martha.

"Settle down please, be calm," I said while gently helping her to the chair.

While motioning for her to sit, I noticed that her dress was wet. I did not want to mention anything at that point. Her face was masked with humiliation and that further triggered her tears, a sign that she was helpless about whatever was on her mind.

"Be calm. I understand, you are safe here," I reassured her.

"He died. Last year ... a day after he turned nine," Maureen continued. Her face had dried up. "He was the world to me. The only reason that made me brave each day, regardless of the condition I have had to live with."

Sister Martha came in while scrutinizing a patient's clinical record. Maureen stopped talking and stared at me. She was afraid, perhaps also tired of exposing her sorrows to everyone. It was by chance that she found me. But despite her determined hold on her suffering, she wanted to talk, it was itching within her, threatening to explode if not given full vent.

Her husband had left her upon receiving the news that she had fistula. It was a dark period in her life. He had some information about the curse that was fistula. It may have been from the angle of science, and it may have been from societal inclination in the belief that it was witchcraft. Regardless of one's inclination, each belief system had a basic understanding that one effect of fistula was a functionless bladder. The leakages had made their debut on their first night in bed together with the child. Maureen had soaked her husband and their child in urine the entire night.

"He was so furious that he threatened to chase me out of the house," Maureen stated.

But he did not, he was still calculating while weighing his patience about the tragedy that was now his wife. And the final blow came.

"Do you remember ... you advised him that I needed six months after the surgery to fully recover?" Maureen looked at me to confirm that I remembered.

My memory on many things about her other than that I helped her deliver safely, were scanty. I nodded my head so as not to disappoint her. However, that was a piece of advice that many husbands never cared to follow. It disturbed me after helping in a fistulotomy only for the man to rescind on his promise and demand to sleep with his sick wife. They did not understand. How ignorant could they be? I had wished that many accompanied their wives to clinic appointments and for counselling as a reminder about how to handle their wives. It was overwhelmingly exhausting to watch a fistula patient who was approaching her healing, start all over again because of a man who could not suppress his lust for six months to allow his partner to recover.

"My husband could not endure that," Maureen continued.

But it was her mother-in-law that fuelled her husband's animosity. She was a heavily-fed woman with a very mean heart. How could she have a daughter-in-law who could not satisfy her son well?

"Now that you are a sickly little thing, what can you help my son with?" she would ask Maureen with a half a sneer on her face.

"Leave her, that one is disabled!" she would tell the son.

That final command from the matriarch was the final blow before her husband's remorseless departure. He did not care that he had once taken the oath, 'for better for worse, in good times and in bad times'.

Sister Martha came in again to remind me that we had a counselling session at the theatre. It was thirty minutes past ten. I begged to leave Maureen for thirty minutes and promised to listen to her to the end.

The counselling sessions were depressing most times. It was difficult to properly attend to those that needed close and constant attention. Our pleas to the administration to allow for the construction of special rooms to place the grieving mothers who had lost their babies often went unanswered. It was unimaginable to soothe and counsel a grieving mother as her peers were overwhelmed by the joys of watching and nursing their newborns.

"Sister, will I ever have a child again?" they would ask, no less than all of them.

"Definitely, and healthy ones too," I would reply, reassuring them, fanning a hope that they were mostly on the verge of losing.

"All my kids will just die like this," one woman who had had two stillbirths said, tired of her situation.

It was difficult uprooting such beliefs from the ladies' minds. Several stubbornly stuck to the idea that once the first child came out as a stillbirth, the rest would also follow. This belief was widespread in the community.

I rushed back to the office after forty minutes to find Maureen still seated, her head was however buried in her hands. She had again wet the seat she was on and feared to raise her face. Nobody ever taught us how to handle embarrassing situations while out in the public. I suspected that she had entertained the thought of running away but the idea was quickly checked by the reality of exposing herself and her situation to strangers who would not want to understand her struggles. It was prudent to organize and have her change clothing to avoid the discomfort and humiliation. Luckily, I had my home clothes which I normally wore to work then switched to my work uniform. I gave them to her.

"This is what I go through every time, it is exhausting … people no longer want to be around me," Maureen continued and broke down.

I witnessed it every day in my line of duty. The pain and loneliness of those women motivated me daily on the project which I had been sitting on about the urgency of creating awareness about fistula out there. The stigma around it heightened the spiral of silence, with many choosing not to talk about their condition to their family or friends around them. Nobody wanted to be near a stinking woman. It was terrible. The social discrimination was particularly harsh on them.

"Why didn't you come for surgery early enough?" I asked her.

She was shocked that I could ask her such a question when her outward appearance bore the unmistakable prints of financial strain.

"Mama was trying to put some funds together but she passed on too," Maureen said, trying hard to conceal the pain in her voice but it broke me too. With her husband having already bolted, and without a job or friends or family, her mother was the only one she had apart from her son. And it was disturbing that the only two people that loved and accepted her in her situation had passed on. Navigating society in search of jobs while carrying the odour everywhere was akin to carrying a placard on one's head labelled 'Do Not Employ Me' while seeking employment. It was what many in Maureen's situation went through.

"I was devastated," she continued. All the little money that she had managed to gather had to be expended on the burial ceremonies. There was no money to seek medical intervention and nobody to turn to. It reaffirmed my judgment about her smile when she greeted me that morning. It was one that had seen all sides of suffering and despair. Such occurrences reminded me of the urgent need to pool resources with the one goal of eradicating obstetric fistula. It was heartbreaking to watch beautiful young girls and women ravaged by fistula, something that could be prevented or treated early. But for the lack of money and information and the fear to talk, they suffered in silence. Suicide was a common option for many of them, who could no longer shoulder the heavy burden of humiliation and rejection, especially by their closest circles of friends and family.

"And what has brought you here today?" I asked Maureen.

"I do not know; I am in pain…" she said while she shyly pointed at an area near her abdomen.

"I do not have anywhere else to go, or anyone to talk to …" As she continued, I moved closer to inspect the painful part she had pointed to with my clinical eye. It was a huge abdominal mass that was also the cause of the odour. Maureen looked at me with hope, mixed with unnamed fear. She did not know what to expect or whether she would be helped or left to die with her pain and troubles. She had grown to mistrust everyone and everything; a consequence of rejection by those she trusted the most. It did not make her feel exceptionally better that she was in hospital. Nobody really cared about her. It was the message her face expressed, painting the picture that she had surrendered to the painful idea that she was worthless and beyond help.

It had been a week of only breaking bad news to many patients I interacted with: death, a terminal illness, a medical complexity that would require a more advanced hospital with the resources ... I was losing my mind. It was depressing. But the feeling I felt upon seeing Maureen break into tears when I broke the news about the free fistula camp was one that I will never get over. She was in disbelief. This is not happening, she must have thought. But her tears bespoke her faith in the surgery and the care she was yet to receive. It made me break too, tears fell from both our eyes. We hugged firmly. Both of us needed the hug.

Mettle

She must be carrying twins, I told myself. The woman had a calm yet poisonous look. I had a strange feeling about her that I could not explain. I had no memory of such a feeling in my fifteen years of nursing experience.

I explained to her that the horizontal positioning of the baby often made it difficult to conduct normal delivery. But I had more depressing news for her that shattered my heart. I hated that I was always the one who informed them. The images of their broken and shocked faces would replay in my head for a very long time. I would have nightmares at times. Losing a child in the last hours of pregnancy was a mortal blow to a mother; one that would be impossible to forget.

"It did not make it," I mentioned.

"What did not make it?" she asked with a tired face.

"The little one," I replied.

It was always important to let out the news to the mother as soon as possible. Her first reaction was strange laughter. While in the state of shock, some are numbed into silence, no longer aware of what is happening to them. Others may break into sudden laughter, confusedly and in disbelief. I figured Ann was one of those that received shocking news with a strange laugh. Laughing at the impossibility of the action.

It would however shock me when she turned to me and claimed that I should produce her child alive as she was. "You shall give me my Martha, alive as she was." She raised her voice into a hysterical siren that pierced deep into my ears. Ann had already named her child Martha, whom she believed we were hiding from her. I had witnessed many silently curse and blame the nurses for causing the death of their children. However, Ann's case was strange. She boldly and loudly announced that I must have done something fishy to her Martha.

I had never handled drama that was that extreme. I gathered my words and passionately appealed to her to calm down.

"You also developed fistula," I tried to inform her despite the chaotic noise all over. But her hysterics were over the roof. Her eyes darted from side to side, filled with tears and the evident pain that she harboured, despite the denial of the death of her child.

"Fistula! You have given me fistula too, you witch!" she cursed.

Ann was suffering from an extreme meltdown. We had to put her to sleep, hoping that she would wake up more accommodative of the death of her child. I thought of separating her and putting her in a more private room, but there was no extra room. It was difficult for those that lost their children to mingle with those who delivered successfully. The cries of the other babies dug grave wounds in the minds of those bereaved. It was practically impossible to console them in those congested rooms that could equally not allow privacy.

When Ann woke up, she was quiet but evidently still in shock. However, the sight of nurses triggered her wails again. She went into an offensive, throwing all manner of curses to the nurses. Ann refused to be consoled. She demanded to see her child. Her wails shot through my heart. I could conceive her pain. Seemingly, it was her first close death in her life, or she may have attached so much emotion and hope to the child that it was almost impossible that something bad would ever happen to her. I could not get around those thoughts to her reality.

It was a delicate moment when Ann further refused to be counselled. She had declined all efforts to console or talk to her. Like a deranged fellow, she would stare at the ceiling for extended periods of time, only breaking to curse afresh when she regained her voice that would frequently fade due to consistent cries. There were matters that one must accept, for such is life. But Ann was not prepared to let go or accept it.

I would witness many other cases like Ann's though of a lesser magnitude. And they would still shatter me. They would gnaw at me. I would watch young mothers, especially those that had not yet handled any major pain or loss in the world, break and disintegrate. Their images and their cries would keep me up at night. Severally, I would contemplate quitting the nursing profession. I would not wake up to the many painful cries and sick faces that reminded me of how terrible life was. How unfortunate it was to be born in poverty. I would not have to watch the many patients rot away in their graves due to sickness, trivial and preventable diseases for lack of a proper medical cover. Yet, I could not bring myself to quit. It would be betrayal to humanity. It would be betrayal to the many women ravaged and mauled and humiliated by fistula when they could prevent or treat it. At times, those cries of loss and heartbreaking stories of women with fistula would remind me of my duty. They would foster my resolve to battle the monster. To save and encourage the young and hopeless girls that despite a series of stillbirths, they could still get a child that would live to give them grandchildren.

I had just reported to my new workstation in Kisumu after a wave of transfers in the medical field. Adapting to new places always triggered fits of anxiety in me. It is always difficult to leave a place you have very deep roots of attachment – memories. This transfer particularly gave me panic attacks I had never had in my life. I was afraid of forming new relationships. I was terrified of getting lost, of not knowing where to get this and that. I was excessively nervous at my new workplace. It sickened me to think that I would not see my husband every evening.

A middle-aged woman was brought in suffering great abdominal pains. Whoever brought her disappeared into oblivion. The woman in travail hinted that she was brought by a stranger and she had no idea who he was. I assumed that he may have imagined he would be forced to cater for the necessary hospital bills and thought it wise to save himself the trouble. I had witnessed many such cases. A Good Samaritan would bring in an accident victim but then disappear to avoid any further obligation that may arise concerning the wounded victim.

The woman looked tired – emotionally and mentally worn out. Her outward appearance gave all signs that she had given up all hope of ever finding happiness. She had surrendered every womanly effort about self-care. It was a similar pattern of suffering and pain or loss. I was only curious about what her story might be.

As I checked her temperature and administered to her pain relievers while conducting the necessary tests, I tried to set her tongue rolling. She was reluctant. Perhaps too tired to talk about herself. Life no longer had any meaning for her. It was pointless and colourless. Despite her condition, she had an erratic temper. Inner pain in a patient would always make them erratic. But my deep intuition directed me to a pain beyond that which she felt physically. It was an affliction of her spirit. Poor woman.

"What is your name?" I asked her.

She failed to reply and shot me an arrogant glance. I was patient with her and asked her the second time, more calmly.

"Mogire," she responded

"Your full name please?"

She shot me another rude glance, as though I was irritating her. She deliberately paused for a while before replying, "Ann Mogire Chunyo."

As I filled in her records, I heard her try to stifle a curse word, and I turned to look. Urine was dripping to the floor from her thighs. Her face folded again angrily. Anger was her way of masking her embarrassment and inner pain. She would repulse any curious eye on her and her situation with a haughty eye and angry face. With that as her defence mechanism, one would feel too intimidated to continue studying her closely. I was not particularly triggered by anything else other than her urine situation. I stated, more so without any cause, "We have interacted before."

"I know!" she replied haughtily.

Her answer fired up my curiosity. By her way of reply, she had admitted to having met me previously. I glanced at her name for several minutes, but it did not register that we had actually met before. I glanced at her from the side, trying to conjure up her memory, but I struggled unsuccessfully.

"You helped me deliver a dead child some years ago in Kisii," she said, possibly after witnessing my struggle trying to remember but too proud to ask again.

The images rushed back to mind and I was baffled. It could not be Ann! What had life done to her? I was doubly curious. Her bulkiness had been washed away, by the turbulence of life perhaps, her round face was now pointed and emotionless apart from her deliberate anger.

"I have lost three children … stillbirths!" she continued, as if talking to herself. She did not need questions for her to relate her story. Her tone had no indication that she deserved any pity. She wanted none, but to tell her story for its own sake.

"The fistula you people gave me has caused me great pain," Ann added, still playing the blame game, only without the hysterics and the violent abuse.

"Have you ever sought treatment?" I asked, ignoring the jibe.

"With what money?" she replied, her tone rising.

"I am tired; in this life, I have already had enough. I do not want any treatment. I now want to rest," she added, almost speaking to herself again as though I was not in the room or I did not matter.

Many of the suicidal cases would often use the word 'rest' to indicate their desire to die. In death, they said, they would find peace. But Ann did not want to talk about the specifics of her story with fistula. Her innate arrogance and pride did not allow her to spill tears all over and pity herself. But, her desire to rest had betrayed that pride. She had suffered just as the many women with fistula had suffered. She had been humiliated by her friends, people close to her and possibly abandoned too. Ann had her silent moments when she would break down and wish things were different, and life would be back to what it was before she suffered fistula. Yet, her mouth could not admit that to strangers, to humans whom she had lost trust in.

"Does your family know you are here?" I asked deliberately to open up her family tale.

"What family? Didn't I tell you I was brought by a stranger?" she shot back angrily.

Her anger was not directed at me, but her absent family. The kin that could not endure her urine stink and her series of stillbirths.

"They imagine that I am cursed. Curse them!" Ann spat, almost to herself again, slowly dropping the guard on her taciturn nature. The way to handle Ann, as I realised, was not to ask her questions. She wanted to be in charge and feel in control. She would talk when she wanted to, possibly listening to the silent questions that ran through my mind. She kept breaking, disintegrating, shedding off her hard exterior. I could see a tear drop. I feared that she would get hysterical again, and I would not be able to handle her. But she did not. Too many sad and cruel events in her life had turned her into stone, though a stone that would shed tears at some point. She would then break completely and beg, "If only I could stop this – these leakages, this humiliation ...." She was begging to be helped, I could not stop the tears myself. Her pain was too deep, and her begging was desperate. It broke me. We both needed help, I thought.

Later that day, I pulled myself together and asked her if I could plan for a counselling session which was available at the hospital support centre. She obliged. She was happy to have a counsellor who would walk with her through this emotional journey to full recovery.

Epilogue

Fistula is one of the conditions that can easily be looked at as unjust and unfair. To begin with, women, who are a vulnerable population in every sense within the African setting, assume the biggest burden when it comes to the condition. Their pain is not limited to what happens to them physically, but also extends to their psychological domain and home environment. While intervention mechanisms are gaining ground across the continent, the fact remains that the level of concern is not proportional to the problem, and this can be deduced from the amount of energy put into matters of policies, funding, awareness and other mitigation measures regarding Obstetric Fistula.

Having dealt with more than 4,000 patients experiencing fistula and stillbirth, we are convinced that we would have had to deal with far fewer cases if the situation was taken a little more seriously by society. Many questions continue to linger in our minds. We have asked ourselves whether the next generation of nurses and doctors will deal with the same issues we deal with. In any case, we are dealing with the same issues doctors and nurses of the previous generation dealt with. There seems to be no end in sight, or is there?

Perhaps the space for awareness is more expanded today than before, but we cannot attach this expansion to direct measures taken by relevant institutions towards cleaning up the backlog of fistula cases. On the contrary, it is possible that growth in other sectors such as ICT with regard to access to mobile phones, computers, as well as internet penetration, have had a larger impact on the general awareness of fistula and stillbirth. Today, information is a click away and those that have access to the internet are closer to disabusing the entrenched views, myths and misconceptions. Those without access to the internet form a large part of the population in Africa. This means that the problem is not about to go away soon, unless deliberate action is guaranteed at every level of society.

Waiting on governments to act may bring forward impractical timelines against a problem whose consequences are almost always imminent. Governments have long proven that their priorities are dictated by what are considered to be public issues. In the African sense, fistula is a personal difficulty and this goes for stillbirth too. They simply do not meet the threshold for public interest, apparently. This is the most underwhelming explanation we feel can be used to sanitize the situation at the government level. It is also why we believe that any large-scale intervention measure must start from the community as the sole solution provider and instead include governments as one of the entities that can be looked at for a solution. But for how long can women wait?

This book has further relied on first-hand information from people who have experienced fistula for years, and whose stories we hope will go a long way in highlighting the fistula burden to the world in a way that has not been seen before. It is impossible to solve something that you do not understand, because in the first place, you have no idea what it is and the gravity it holds as an issue. For this reason, there is almost no better starting point, we believe, than research, whose overarching objective will be pegged on the need to ground solutions that transcend any change of governments across Africa.

It is a difficult place to be a doctor dealing with these kinds of cases. Yet it is also fulfilling to know that you are giving back life to someone whose problems have defined them for as long as they have been battling the condition. However, not having to deal with preventable cases is a far much better position than having to deal with them.

We, therefore, hope that our readers drink our passion and join the conversation that will help bring to an end a chapter that should never have been written for the African women. In the end, we hope that the reader will grow a desire for action which will stimulate their involvement in intervention programmes that will retain lifelong impact for individuals and communities.

Author's note

I have had the privilege of treating patients, mostly women, from all walks of life. As a doctor, it is possible, I have realized, to be convinced that what you do every day is work. Certainly, you are paid for what you do, but is it really work? That is the question that for a long time has served as a reminder of the kind of doctor I want to define myself as. The conclusion I have arrived at after many years of service is that what we do is more than simply work: it is community service. Many doctors, I am sure, will agree with me on that. A lot more, especially those that interact with vulnerable groups such as women, will agree even more.

It is difficult for the sight of a suffering woman to leave your mind. In Africa, women are the pride of the community. It is through them that the continuity of the society is guaranteed. The shame of this statement is the fact that in spite of this high level of reverence for women, they suffer some of the most avoidable problems. It is not only medical complexities that they have to deal with, they also have to deal with socially-generated issues that have everything to do with labelling them negatively and using that same label as a tool to victimize them.

Obstetric fistula and stillbirth are not more of women's problems than they are community issues. We have, in our own making, chosen to label them women's issues, yet in between the occurrence of both conditions, men are involved. It is this labelling that results in the social issues that these women face, which only serve to add to their tribulations.

While the problem of the society needs an urgent intervention, which I am convinced starts and ends with the creation of widespread awareness on the condition, the medical side of it also requires a lot of re-thinking, if not an overhaul.

There are many improvised ways healthcare workers apply to deal with these cases. We need, however, to move away from improvisation and head towards structure. Structure is what will provide a uniform and standardized approach, which will ensure optimum outcomes. Many policy documents have been crafted towards this end, except that they remain dusty forgotten papers, hidden away from the implementation progress. It is important that they are dusted, updated and put in the pipeline for action.

One of the issues that I am persuaded is a weak link is, as has been reflected in a number of the narrations in this book, the communication channels that are meant to support both fistula care and matters surrounding stillbirth. A good example is why in this century, we still do not have proper referral structures for patients in many African countries. This is a two-pronged issue that includes referrals between different departments in the same hospital and referrals from one hospital to another. In both cases, it is not unusual to see a patient stuck, attempting to explain complex medical terms that they have no hold of to another doctor when it would simply be much easier to hand over a report written by one professional to another. This is an unnecessary burden we bestow on patients.

It is imperative that going forward, we attain ways to profile patients with a fistula as the starting point to establishing predictors of success of fistula surgery in Africa. We must not make it their duty to come forward, but our responsibility to locate them. I have been part of dozens of fistula camps and one of the observations my team and I made was that whenever transport service is provided for those who cannot afford it, many women turn up for the camp compared to when this is not made available. This is a pointer to just how many women with fistula remain out there, hindered from accessing surgery simply because they are not reachable.

If we erect structures that can access them, as has been a great success with contact tracing in the wake of the COVID-19 pandemic, it is possible to put more women out of danger. This calls for bringing together an active data of facility and patient profiles dominated by socio-demographic information: which would include age, education, parity, marital status, occupation, religion, contact details, home/residential address and country of origin. The data could also go as far as accommodating the social characteristics of the patients' spouses and whether or not the said spouses left the relationships because of the fistula problem. Even more elaborately, it would be ideal to have a bank of information about the fistula histories of patients and the symptoms they presented (whether the patient had urine or stool leakage or both), previous repairs and duration of leakage as well as their medical history, menstruation patterns, labour and childbirth characteristics.

Equally, at the pre-operative care level, fistula education and supportive counselling needs to be given on a one-to-one basis for all patients in the ward. It is common, for instance, to find patients who are unwilling to drink the required amount of fluid for fear of increased leakage. This is despite the fact that a high fluid intake is important intra-operatively as it allows for easy identification of the ureters. As part of the personalized education to the patients, this information must first be made available to them as the beginning point of inducting them into the understanding of what they need to do when it comes to fistula care.

As the goal shifts towards intra-operative care, the guiding surgical principle which has been evidenced by multiple studies and which relates to the idea that the first attempt at fistula repair offers the best chance for a successful surgery, must take precedence in the mindset of those charged with the responsibility. This means that one must refer patients when they have the slightest doubt about handling their situation as they will have assessed it. Even before then, upon receiving the patient in theatre, healthcare providers must build a means to make them comfortable and settled during psychotherapy.

The immediate post-operative care is also one stage that must not be ignored. Any complications noted during this stage should be dealt with urgently and the care extended from the time the patient leaves theatre until the 7th post-operative day. Healthcare workers must also prepare beforehand for anticipated complications that may include catheter blockage and stress incontinence. All complications that will be observed after surgery and soon after the patient leaves theatre must, importantly, be documented and included in the patient's report, which must be shared with the patient as well as kept alive in the hospital records in case of future need.

What is often overlooked and which I prefer to conclude my note with, is the critical phase that is long-term follow-up and visitation that is part of post-operative care. While short-term follow up visits to the patients could span about two weeks after discharge, long-term follow up visits must be initiated from four weeks post-surgery.

The idea behind this phase is to assess fistula closure and associated complications. Post-operatively, a dye test should be done for every patient at week two to help the surgeon in assessing fistula closure and continence, and where necessary, removal of the urethral catheter.

Therefore, looking ahead, the future for Africa's interaction and care for women with fistula is not in the hands of a special unseen saviour, but in ourselves, our institutions and our ability to comprehend that this is not a by-the-way problem; it is a real issue that has to be addressed by any means necessary.

Printed in the United States
by Baker & Taylor Publisher Services